The A-Z of Parenting: Babies

by Sienna's Mum

First paperback edition 2022

Book design by Publishing Push
Illustrations by Kerri Cunningham (Murphy's Sketches)

978-1-80227-670-1 (paperback)
978-1-80227-671-8 (ebook)

This book is dedicated to my daughter,
Sienna. The girl with the big smile,
my ray of sunshine.

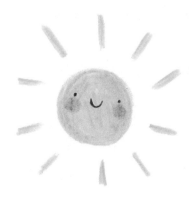

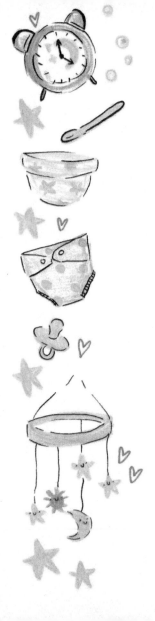

contents

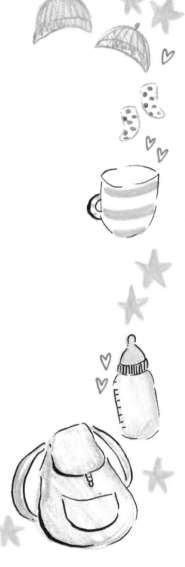

Acknowledgements

During the first year of Sienna's life, I learnt so much about babies. I was fortunate to be able to go to 2-3 baby groups a week and so spent a lot of time with babies and their mums. It was really great to talk, share experiences, and have the support of a tribe of other mums as we navigated our way through being new parents. I am forever grateful for this network as well as the baby class leaders who gave endless energy to entertain our babies and who offered support, advice, and shared experiences which have been invaluable.

It was also during this first year that I spent many weeks in therapy, and so it wouldn't be right to not pass acknowledgement to my therapist for keeping me sane and level-headed during a time of great uncertainty. Even though I didn't tell anyone I was writing this book, as I am a firm believer in working hard in silence and letting the outcome do the talking, I wouldn't be the person I am today without the friends and family who have been along for the ride too, so here is your shout out. The people who have truly been there, you know who you are, so thank you.

If through this book, I can impart just half of the wonderful pieces of wisdom I have been so lucky to receive, then the readers who have most likely skipped this page are in for a treat.

About me

My name is Emma and I am Sienna's mum. A proud first time mum who is unapologetically obsessed with the little bundle of joy who came into our world. Although I have aimed to write the following A-Z tips in a fairly objective manner, a little of who I am and the experiences I have learned from have naturally come into play. So it's only fair that you know a bit about who is giving you these tips.

As well as being a mum to Sienna, I am passionate about sustainability and the environment. Having graduated from University in 2011 with a First Class Bachelor of Science degree, I have since worked in Corporate Social Responsibility for over 10 years. I'm also a qualified yoga instructor with the British Wheel of Yoga and have a meditation podcast in the making, ready to share a calm moment with you.

I am the type of person who, when working on any given task gives it my all. This did not change when I had a baby. I saw it as my duty and new full time career to learn everything there is to know about parenting a baby.

Introduction

So, you are having a baby. Or you have had a baby. Or you know it all and need someone else to learn a thing or two (and if you are that 'someone else' reading this, then please do not take offence- nobody is born knowing this stuff!) Which, let's face it there is a lot of stuff we have found ourselves needing to know.

This little book aims to give you the heads up on a few things that I have learnt along the way, or that I have found myself wishing I already knew. People say babies do not come with instruction manuals, well consider this as close as it can get.

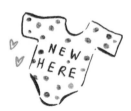
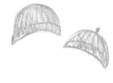

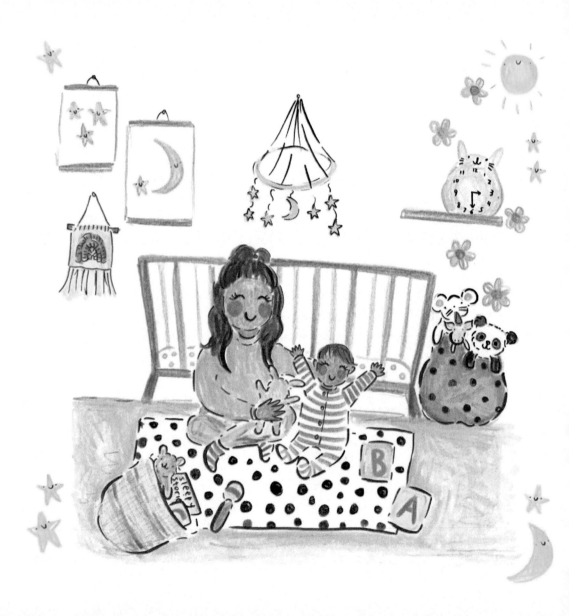

1. Awake windows

It's worked out quite well that this fits in with the first chapter because it's a biggie! Sleep, ah who remembers that? I remember naively stating when my baby was a few weeks old, that if not sleeping was the hardest part of having a baby, that it was going to be easy. Fast forward a few months and I could completely understand why sleep deprivation is used as a form of torture. It's hard! We need sleep to function, to regulate our emotions, and for our brains to be at least half switched on! If like me, you bought books to read up on how to sleep train your baby, then feel free to read them (pretty cool if you have time) but remember that every baby is different (see chapter 5), that depending on their age babies will likely not be developmentally able to sleep 'through the night' which technically only means 5 hours anyway (I know!), and that you can according to neurological schools of thought cause babies harm by allowing them to 'cry it out'. I'm not here to judge, you know your baby better than anyone else in the world, but if you are interested in finding out more about this then check out some research into the correlation between cortisol and brain development. Then when you are ready to encourage your baby to sleep more, without 'training', this is where holistic sleep methods come into play! Cue, awake windows (also referred to as wake windows but that wouldn't work with the A!).

Awake windows refer to the maximum awake time that your baby can handle during the day before it becomes sensible to encourage them into a nap. This is important, because if babies don't get enough sleep in during the day then they can become overtired and this can negatively impact their sleep during the night. Thought tiredness meant more sleep? Not necessarily! Let's cut to the chase, wondering how many hours we are talking about? This is where it is a little harder, because there is no one-size fits all model (sorry!). Awake windows change with your baby's age. However, if you follow the table below you are onto a winner:

Age	Awake Window
0 – 1 month	40 minutes
1 – 2 months	40 – 60 minutes
2 – 3 months	60 – 75 minutes
3 – 4 months	60 – 90 minutes
4 – 6 months	75 – 105 minutes
6 – 8 months	2 – 2.5 hours
8 – 10 months	2 – 3.5 hours
10 – 12 months	2 - 4 hours

At first it can be hard to encourage your baby to nap at the right interval since their last wake, especially depending on what age your baby is when you start following awake windows. However, rest assured that after a few weeks, putting your baby down for a nap will be easier. Nap lengths will vary, and this will depend on a number of factors such as sleep cycles, babies age, their sleep needs, growth spurts, developmental appropriateness etc. My point here is to encourage you to focus not on the length of the nap, nor even the time of day since technically babies can't tell the time, but simply to focus on the length of time your baby is awake in between naps. In my experience, you can forget about everything else- and use the spare time to recycle those sleep training books.

Incidentally, it also doesn't matter 'how' you send your baby to sleep either. Don't get caught up in rules about putting babies in their cribs or cots awake, half awake, drowsy but not asleep etc. Feed your baby to sleep if you want (I still do this), and don't feel guilty either. Particularly if you breastfeed it can be reassuring to know that breastfeeding your baby to sleep, as well as for comfort, is a completely natural as well as developmentally appropriate thing to do. Mammals have been feeding their babies to sleep since the beginning of time. Plus believe it or not, feeding your baby to sleep will not mean that you have an 18 year old one day who is incapable of sleeping without a milkshake. Babies and children learn to move into milestones when they are developmentally ready, be it rolling, crawling, talking, or sleeping. We don't force them to learn any other milestones before they are ready, so try not to get influenced into doing this with sleep. If you want to do this, that's fine. My point is merely that this does not benefit the baby or affect their future sleep behaviour.

Awake windows

There are other holistic sleep methods that you can explore as and when you need to, and there is more on this topic in chapter 26. But let's not complicate things when we really don't need to. We have 25 other chapters of things to learn, so for now note down the wake window table and let's move on.

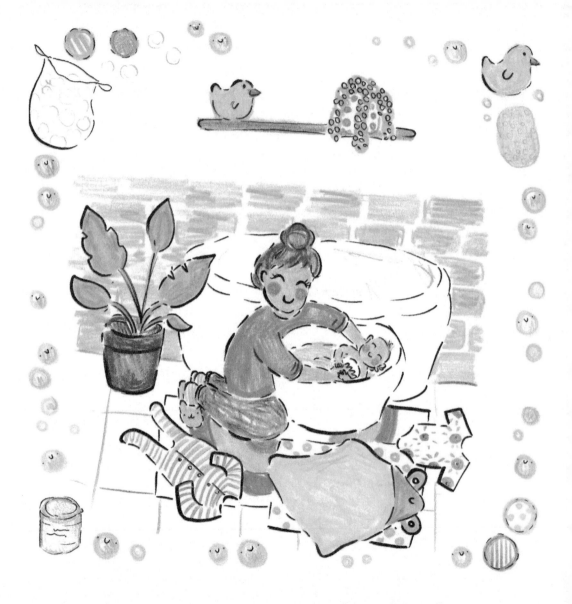

2. Bath time

When you have a brand new, teeny tiny, fragile baby, the thought of giving them a bath can seem a little bit daunting. Preparation is key, so to begin with let us go through the things you will need or may find useful for bathing your babe:

- 2x towels (this will enable you to use one to dry them with, leaving the other for the baby to lie on, so that they won't end up laying on a slightly cold and damp towel). It can be handy for the towel you're drying them with to have a little hood to keep them warm and dry from top to toe.

- Cotton wool or reusable soft cotton pads (these will be used to clean around the eyes and face mostly), for more on reusables see chapter 18.
- Top and tail bowl / baby bath.

In terms of the bath itself, that is really it for now!

Top Tip: If you have all these items in a designated bath time caddy, it will save you time gathering things from various locations ahead of each bath.

You may also want to have the following items nearby to make it an easy and smooth process for you:

- Vest (See chapter 3 for more on clothing)
- Babygrow/sleepsuit
- Clean nappy
- Barrier cream

You might have noticed there has been no mention of any bath products, and this is completely intentional. The soft and perfect skin your baby has is super sensitive too, so avoid any bath products until your baby is at least 4-6 weeks old. Infact, try not to give your baby a bath at all until their umbilical cord has completely fallen off (see chapter 21), and then ideally no more than once a week for the first 6 weeks of their life. This is because the vernix coating (that white, creamy icky stuff) that has surrounded the baby since the third trimester is full of microbial and healing properties. In other words, it's good for them!

The first baths you give your baby, don't need to be 'baths' as such. This is where the top and tail bowls come in. You don't even need a specific top and tail bowl either to be honest, the idea is just to ensure you bathe your baby with separate water for the face and bum (for obvious reasons) and this can be done with two separate regular bowls. When they are in an actual baby bath, you won't need more than about 10cm of water up until around 6 months. The water should be warm, the guidance is 37 degrees but you'll soon know what the temperature of the right water feels like without needing a thermometer, and some baby baths come with built in temperature gauges. Remember, a baby's skin burns and scalds much easier than an adults so keep it cool.

Use the cotton wool pads to spread cooled boiled water around their eyes, making sure you wipe from the inside corner by the top of the nose outwards, and then discard the pad so you don't wipe dirt back through the eye. It kind of goes without saying, but use a separate cotton pad for each eye too! You'd be surprised how easily babies can get eye infections. You can also use the

cotton pads to wash behind the ears, neck and hands using warm water–
which once you've got the hang of doing, are all areas that will be quick and
easy to wash daily.

In terms of frequency, there's no need to bath your baby everyday until they
are around 6 months old (and weaning, aka getting very messy on a daily
basis- see chapter 23). However, establishing a bedtime routine can help with
sleep and I've really found it helpful to bath Sienna every evening before bed
for this reason (see chapter 26). I mean, who doesn't find a bath relaxing?!

There are lots of risks with babies, many of which are covered under chapter
15 but it's important to note here that drowning is one of the most common
causes of child death. All it takes is 5cm (2inches) of water, and it's often silent.
That's not intended to scare you, but just to make you aware of this very real,
and common risk.

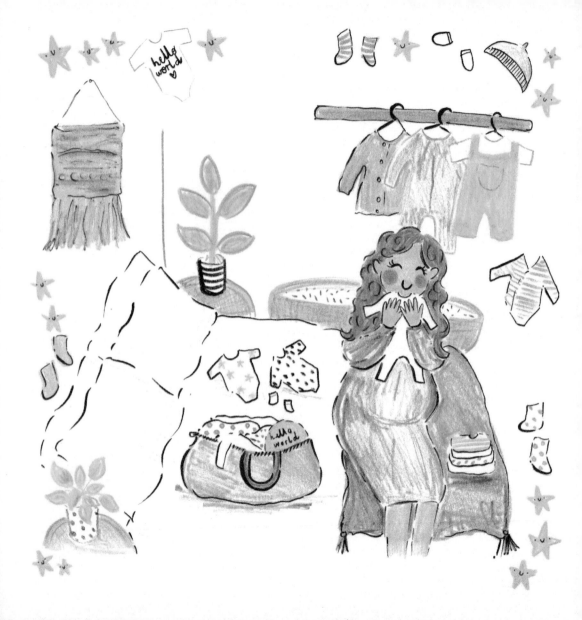

3. clothes

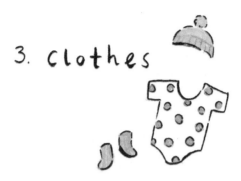

This chapter is all about dressing your little one. Buying baby clothes can be fun and there are so many cute outfits out there, which means a lot of different styles and options too. This chapter aims to give you the heads up on what to dress your baby in depending on things such as the temperature and time of day, as well as offer some practical tips on making clothes easy to wear. Not forgetting the all important hospital bag, and the baby clothes that will be useful to have on hand from day dot.

Let's start from the beginning, the hospital bag! I remember packing Sienna's hospital bag like it was yesterday. I'd washed her new clothes (not essential, but if you combine the potential germs and chemicals from the production with a mum in the nesting phase it felt right), ironed them (I have no sane explanation that can help to justify this other than it was so cute to see the tiniest of clothes on the ironing board), and hung them in her nursery. Now, when it came to selecting which items to pack for the hospital bag, I only knew what friends had suggested might be useful. Some were, and some weren't, and I also found identifying them in the hospital confusing when I had several other things going on after having had a pretty traumatising labour. So here's a handy list of what you may find useful to pack, and why!

 Vests
Long or short sleeves depending on the season/temperature- these go underneath the babygrows (which may be obvious to some, but I didn't know this until the midwives told me in the hospital that Sienna needed a vest under her outfit!)

 Babygrow (also referred to as a sleepsuit)
Your baby can wear this all day and night on top of the vest.

 Hat
Not all babies need a hat after birth. The theory is that your little one will have been born from a cosy warm environment, and the hat may help them to feel snug and warm again. However, the days of

insisting they are essential are gone and some schools of thought have even suggested against them. You could pack one to be on the safe side, but you also don't need to panic if you haven't got one.

 Teeny tiny gloves

These are generally useful to help to stop your baby from scratching themselves. Or if you find yourself with a jaundice baby who has to undergo phototherapy / light treatment, the gloves will help. That thought seems a bit random I know, but bear with me on this one! Sienna and I were in hospital for 5 days after her birth due to various factors, jaundice being one of them. During the phototherapy, babies have to wear an eye mask for protection. Sienna hated wearing this and would try her hardest to take it off, and the gloves proved invaluable in preventing her from being successful in her mission. Checkout the sleepsuits you've got too though, as some of them come with built in gloves that you can tuck over the hands as and when required. These are great because the separate gloves can get lost and fall off pretty easily which makes them slightly less practical.

 Packing cubes/bags

These can be used to separate items and label them accordingly, which helps when you need to find things fast in the chaos.

That's really all you need in terms of clothing. Take a few of each and you're good to go.

When you're home, a vest and babygrow/sleepsuit is all you really need. A long sleeve vest in the winter months, a short sleeve vest in the summer, and the babygrow/sleepsuit on top. With a few of these set aside you'll be well equipped.

At night time, sleeping bags are a safe option for bedding. You can use the table below to help identify which tog sleeping bag, and whether to opt for long or short sleeve vests under their sleepsuit at night. Bear in mind that babies can't regulate their temperatures in the way that we can. This is why it's important to prevent them getting too hot or too cold. However, don't become obsessed with the table below either, as you'll soon learn what works and doesn't work for your baby. So this is just a guide:

Nursery Temperature	Sleeping Bag	Vest	Sleepsuit
>26 degrees celsius	Not required	Short sleeved	Not required
24 – 25 degrees celsius	0.5 tog	Short sleeved	Not required
22 – 23 degrees celsius	1 tog	Short sleeved	Yes
18 – 21 degrees celsius	1 tog / 2.5 tog	Long sleeved / short sleeved	Yes
15 – 17 degrees celsius	2.5 tog	Long sleeved	Yes
<15 degrees celsius	3.5 tog	Long sleeved	Yes

The last thing I wanted to cover when it comes to clothing, is more of a practical top tip to help make dressing your baby easier. Clothes that button up at the back can be less comfortable for the little one, and also be a little more awkward for you when it comes to buttoning them up. This is because when they are new, and you're new to them, the easiest position for your baby to be in for outfit changes is lying on their back.

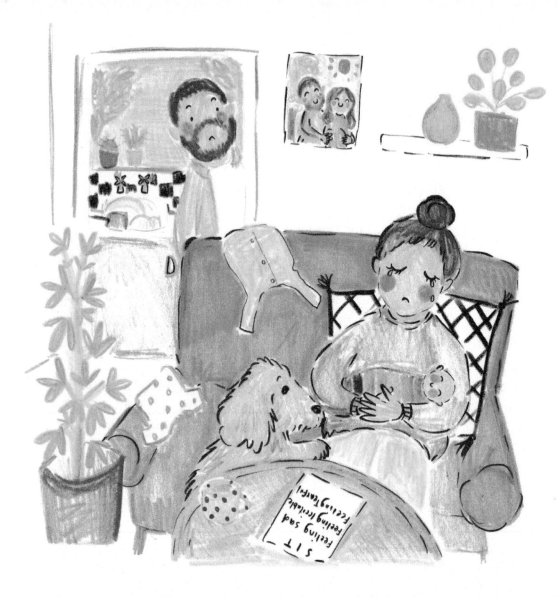

4. Depression and Anxiety

Having a baby is the hardest job in the world. It's also the most rewarding and wonderful time of your life. The juxtaposition of the two can run in parallel and finding it hard doesn't take away from the love you have for your baby, nor how much you adore being a parent. When you have a baby everything changes from the dynamic of your relationship with your partner, as well as that of your friendships and relationships with family (see chapter 9 for more on families, and 10 on jealousy). Your whole life turns upside down and it can often feel as though your life isn't 'yours' anymore. You may no longer be able to do the things you once did so freely, without lots of planning, or even at all depending on the level of support system you have in place. As well as this, you may have been used to having certain coping mechanisms for life up until this point, and now you might be unable to access them due to having a 24 hour job keeping a baby alive and well. As an example, pre baby I would visit my local hot yoga studio at least twice a week. I didn't realise how much I depended on the ability to do this to keep me sane, until it was something I was no longer able to access.

For some of you, this may not apply, but I found myself bringing up a baby and feeling very alone. I had people in my life who would come and see me and the baby, but none who would really help. Then there's the consideration that when we have a new baby, the type of help we want may differ. Let's talk about Primary Maternal Preoccupation, something very real and pretty normal but perhaps not discussed very much. The best way for me to describe Primary Maternal Preoccupation is that it's the obsessive, almost animal instinct behaviour of a mother. Have you ever heard people talk about how in the midst of the night, no matter how long they've been asleep for (although let's face it, it's probably not long with a baby around), they would wake up to the lightest of sounds from their baby? This is a real thing! I'm the type of person who pre baby, would have had 5 alarms set for the morning and would manage to subconsciously snooze each of them several times before needing a physical elbow from my other half to wake up. When I was pregnant, we even joked that this would become a concern when Sienna was born- how would I wake up when I'm such a deep sleeper? Cue a heightened sense of awareness like nothing you have ever experienced before. The most natural, out of your control, state of being whereby you will be blinkered to the care of your baby over and above anything else. Quite literally, at the expense of all else too. This for many mothers will also mean that you don't want anyone to hold your baby, so the offers of help will be worthless and often make you feel worse because it just reminds you that not a single sole can really help. The feeling of being isolated and exhausted, but not being ready for anyone to step in is a difficult reality. The anxious feeling in your stomach when someone is holding your baby, the baby who not so long ago was that literal feeling in your stomach. The anger when someone snatches your baby from your arms (please don't ever do this to a new mum, I am speaking from experience when I say it's not helpful and it is not okay!) These feelings are all part and parcel of being a new mum. Being comfortable with other people caring for your baby can be a long road, and I just want everyone reading this to know that this is normal. If you're the dad who's partner won't let you out of sight because she needs eyes on the baby at all times, just know it's not personal! If you're the mum who is feeling all sorts of feels, just know that it does and will get easier. You'll even enjoy having a little bit of time to yourself at some point, which may seem hard to believe when you're in the middle of it but trust me on this. Feeling isolated and exhausted can quickly lead to resentment and feelings of sadness, but I hope it helps to know this is a normal phase and that like all phases it will pass.

If you are able to ask for help from those around you, perhaps consider asking for help with jobs around the house as this can help to lift the burden without adding to anxiety. If the anxiety does however start to take over and lead to low mood or depression, the general advice is to talk to a GP, midwife or health visitor so that you can access support. From my experience, speak to your GP and ask for a referral for talking therapy. Postnatal depression is very common and can crop up at any point within the first year of your baby being born.

Feeling Sad?
Feeling Irritable?
Feeling Tearful?

Time to S-I-T down and do something about it.

There are also services you can call or text for support if this is more accessible for you. In the UK, these are good numbers to have to hand:

- Call 116 123 to talk to Samaritans, or email: jo@samaritans.org for a reply within 24 hours
- Text "SHOUT" to 85258 to contact the Shout Crisis Text Line, or text "YM" if you're under 19.

Under 19's can also call 0800 1111 to talk to Childline . The number will not appear on your phone bill.

For urgent advice, and immediate action also know that you can call 111 or 999.

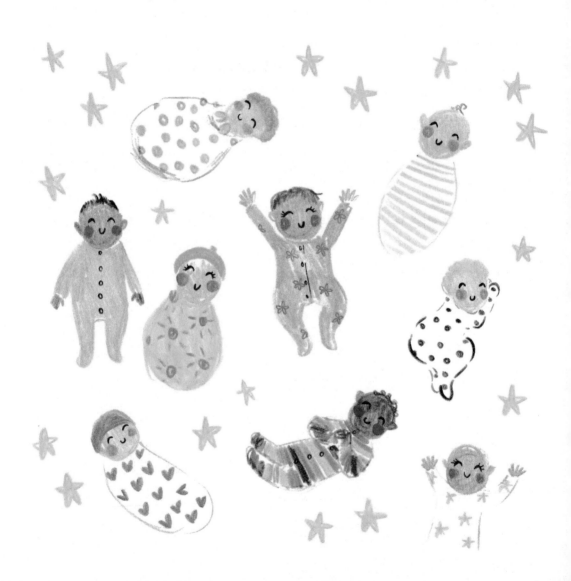

5. Every Baby is Different

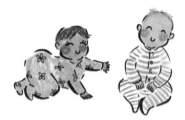

This is a short chapter because the title tells you everything you need to know, though it's important enough to dedicate a chapter to nonetheless. When you have a baby lots of advice will come your way from other people. The advice is with good intention and comes from genuine experiences. However, this does not mean that it will necessarily be relevant or appropriate for your baby, or for you.

The parents who have the baby who sleeps through the night, will want to share what they did. This doesn't mean it will work for your baby.

The parents who have the baby who crawled at 6 months will want to shout from the rooftops that their baby is a genius, it doesn't mean yours isn't.

The parents who let their baby cry it out, and their kids turned out fine, doesn't mean you should automatically consider this method.

We live in a world where access to information is at our fingertips and is available 24/7. There is just so much information and I found this confusing, especially because a lot of it is conflicting! But of course it's conflicting because no single parent on this earth has had the same experience with the same baby. They are all different, as are we. Take Instagram for instance, there are so many accounts run by self proclaimed sleep consultants all sharing different methods. You'll have some insisting that 'Feed-Wake-Sleep' cycles are a proven way to get your baby to sleep, also referred to as 'Eat-Awake-Sleep-You time' (or E.A.S.Y). I look back on the me a few months ago, sleep deprived and naïve, I tried this method. It's a method that moves away from feeding to sleep, yet will approve using a dummy instead. Let's un-pick this shall we, because let's face it neither feeding to sleep nor using an artificial replica of a similar motion for comfort, are representative of a baby falling to sleep independently. It also essentially encourages your baby to go to sleep potentially hungry. I'm not sure if you've ever tried going to sleep on an empty stomach, but compare that to a post Sunday lunch nap and we all know which one led you into a happier, more fulfilled and longer sleep; food comas are real! I've slightly digressed here but my point is that these methods exist (as do holistic sleep methods) and they do work for plenty of mums and babies, but that still doesn't mean it will work or is right for your baby.

Of course, to some extent the only way you'll learn and find out what does work for your baby, is with a little trial and error. The purpose of this chapter is just to remind you that your baby is completely, totally, perfectly unique in every way shape and form. Never listen fully to anything apart from your instinct. Only you know your baby. Be empowered to be their person, the person who stands up for their single needs above all else. Be 'that' parent.

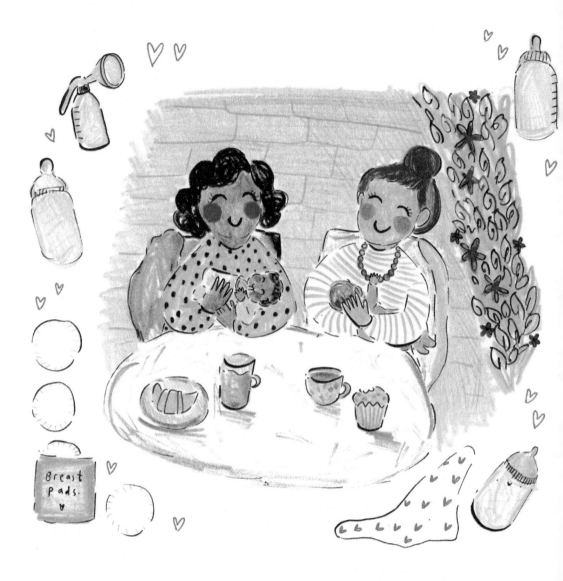

6. Feeding

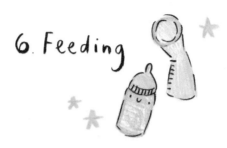

This chapter is all about feeding from ages 0-6 months. After this, it'll be time for weaning and there's a lot on that in chapter 23. For now we're pretty much talking about milk; formula vs breast, including expressing and when it's okay to cry over spilt milk.

Let's start with breastfeeding, for no particular reason other than it comes first alphabetically. Incidentally, I exclusively breastfed Sienna but that doesn't mean breast is always best. As we know from chapter 5, every baby is different. The decision on how to feed your baby initially starts with you, and it's a big decision to make so understanding the pros and cons can really help with your choice.

Learning to breastfeed for the first time, with a new baby who is also learning, can be difficult. You'll be tired from labour, emotional from hormones, and recovering from the birth. As I mentioned in an earlier chapter, Sienna and I were in the hospital for 5 days after her birth due to both the blood loss I had during the birth, and Sienna having jaundice. Although this was overall a pretty traumatising time, I take from it a huge positive in that I had access not only to 24/7 midwifery care, but also the care of specialist feeding nurses. It was through the advice, patience, and kindness of the feeding specialists in particular that my confidence was built enough to get Sienna breastfeeding.

From this experience, it may be useful for you to know that it takes time and that this time may go on even longer if you have a jaundice baby, as they're often too sleepy to feed in the beginning and generally have trouble feeding. During the time that it does take to establish a successful breastfeeding regime, it can be useful to supplement your baby. You can do this with formula, or with harvested colostrum. I didn't harvest any colostrum pre birth but was able to do this from the hospital bed with the syringes provided by the hospital. You can however do this at any time after 36 weeks and freeze it for if/when you need it. If you are wondering how to collect it, it's a manual process which involves essentially squeezing the nipple and collecting each little drop of 'liquid gold' into a syringe. This can be fed to your baby straight from the syringe. For the first 4 days of life, Sienna had a mixture of colostrum and formula to ensure she was putting on weight. During these days, I'd offer the breast using a 'nose to nipple' technique as instructed by the midwives, and manually squeeze out what I could to give her the initial scent / taste but she just wasn't interested. My advice is to keep persisting with this. Just because you've supplemented with formula, doesn't mean you don't have a breastfeeding baby. The day your milk comes in is often the day that the baby will start feeding. What they don't tell you is that you don't always have a milk supply straight away! I didn't know this, and it turns out that my supply was delayed due to the blood I lost in labour. So in hindsight it was always going to take a little longer to establish breastfeeding. I hope that knowing this, offers you some reassurance.

How to hold your baby when breastfeeding is also something important to learn, and there are a few different positions that can work with this. With all of them, it's important to make sure that your baby's neck, shoulders, and back are supported before bringing the baby to your breast. Bringing the baby to you is key so that they can learn to latch themselves, even though it can be tempting to lean forward in order to take your breast to the baby's mouth. When you bring the baby to your breast, you want to aim for their nose to be level with your nipple (you can physically angle your breast to help with this) and then you can let their head tilt back a little which will help to encourage them to open wide. With the baby's chin touching your breast and their nose clear, they may latch on from here. Don't worry if not, from this place you can also try physically pointing the nipple towards their mouth to encourage the baby to learn what to do. It will often take several attempts of this, including some that you think are successful before realising that the baby wasn't actually feeding.

> **Top Tip**: A tip to help identify if the baby is feeding, is to look out for their cheeks which will look fuller and rounded.

When you have established feeding, what you often aren't told is how painful it can be. Invest in a good nipple cream and know that this period of pain doesn't last. After a while, it's pain free I promise.

Expressing milk can be useful, even if you don't plan to introduce a bottle. Breastmilk has so many beneficial purposes so if you are able to store some in the freezer then rest assured it won't go to waste. For example, breastmilk can be used to make ice lollies ready for teething, it can be used to help eye infections and blocked tear ducts, and it is also great in the bath to help treat eczema, acne, nappy rash, cuts and insect bites. When you're weaning your baby too (see chapter 23 for more on weaning), breastmilk can even be added to purees!

If breastfeeding isn't an option for you, formula is your friend. As I mentioned, I had a brief stint at formula feeding whilst learning to breastfeed. There's a whole chapter on sterilising so head to 19 if that's something you're keen to find out more about. For formula feeding, you'll need several bottles, as well as teats (note that teats come in age appropriate sizes), and a bottle brush so that you can clean the bottles prior to sterilising them. You can buy formula as a powder or in a ready-made format. It's a sensible idea to have some of the ready made bottles to hand when your baby is first born in case you need them in the hospital, as powder requires preparation which often isn't possible from the hospital. You may choose to purchase a prep machine for super simple preparation of powder milk for when at home, guaranteeing the perfect temperature for the bottle in 1 minute! These aren't essential and do have some controversy around them, with many health professionals advising against them completely, so my advice is to do your research and decide what is best for you. When it comes to feeding your baby using a bottle, aim to keep the bottle angled horizontally as this helps prevent the baby from taking in too much air by allowing a steady flow.. Generally speaking, formula babies tend to be more windy so just be mindful of this and offer short breaks to wind your baby.

Top Tip: Supplement breastfed babies with vitamin D from birth, and vitamins A, C and D from 6 months.

Babies drinking more than 500ml of formula do not need vitamins, but bear in mind when they move to cows/other milk they are then recommended to take the A, C and D supplements as above until age 5.

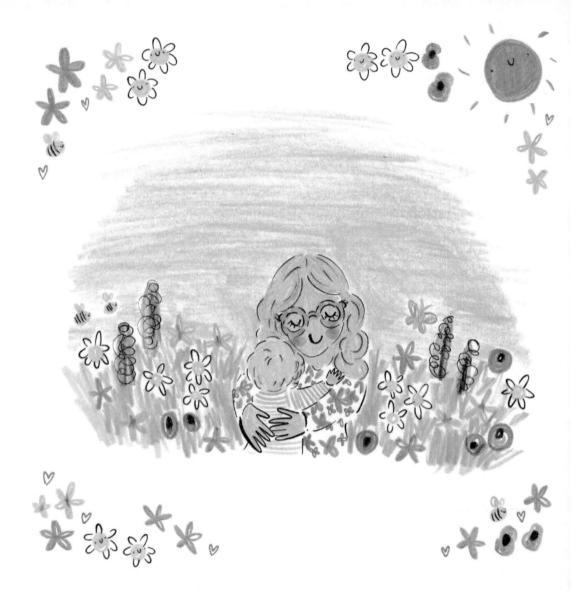

7. Gentle Parenting

I remember when I was about 6 months pregnant, a friend of mine mentioned parenting approaches and I did what I often used to do which is to smile and go along with the conversation but really I had no clue what she was talking about. I got home and ran an internet search about parenting styles, and came across plenty of studies and articles about 4 predominant approaches: authoritative, authoritarian, permissive, and neglectful. This chapter doesn't talk about any of these, and I never did read up on them enough to decide what they were or which one I wanted to follow. Which to be honest worked out quite well for me, as somehow when my daughter was born I fell into what just felt completely natural to me. Without even knowing that it was a thing, I had adopted a 'gentle' parenting approach. I wanted to cover this style of parenting in this book to offer you some food for thought when it comes to considering the type of parental choices you may find yourself making in the upcoming months, and years.

Becoming a parent is one of the most life changing, challenging, and rewarding things you may ever do. We have so much to learn, and our lives will never be the same again. We know we want the absolute best for our little bundle of joy, but what does this really equate to? Here are some what/when/why/who/how questions to ask yourselves. Consider how the answers may help to shape your parenting:

- What did you like and dislike about how your parents raised you?
- What does a happy, confident, successful child look like to you?
- When your child is grown up, what do you want them to be proud of you for?
- When you are older, what do you want to be proud of your grown up child for?
- Why did you decide to have kids?
- Why do you think some people are unhappy (and how can you help to avoid this for your child)?

- Who has helped to shape your values as a person?
- Who do you want your child to be like when they grow up?
- How can you help your partner, based on each other's experiences, strengths and weaknesses?
- How can you be authentic with your child?

The best way I can describe gentle parenting in a nutshell, is that it's the long game. You need a lot of patience (but then which parent doesn't). You'll also need some thick skin when it comes to the views of other people (again, this applies to parenting in general, because not everyone will adopt the same approach as you). But that's okay too, we live and let live- and when the Karen's of the world tell us we're making a rod for our own back we muster enough energy to ignore them somehow.

Gentle parenting means not letting your child sleep from the exhaustion of crying it out, and recognising that babies do things for no reason other than that they are babies, and that this is ok! Even if they've slept through the night before, remember that they are babies, they are meant to be unpredictable. Sometimes it really is just a case of adjusting our expectations and bringing ourselves back to reality. Babies and children need us, and we have a role to play in meeting that need. It's okay to contact-nap, and co-sleep; contrary to what some people may tell you, these aren't creating bad habits. You won't end up with a 20 year old sleeping in your bed.

Gentle parenting means promoting a relationship with your child that is based on a partnership. Encouraging them to make decisions and choices based on their own willingness, as opposed to external pressures which could leave them not really understanding why they are doing something. It's teaching them to do things because of the positive reasons behind them, not through fear of punishment. Because by comforting your child during these times of need, you will be demonstrating empathy- a positive trait that your child will learn.

Gentle parenting means no matter how crazy your 5 year old has got when he/she is really tired one morning and doesn't want to go to school, so much so that they hit out at you and physically punch you in the arm, that you remember children do not have the ability to regulate their emotions or process what it happening. This is a real life example shared to me by an old friend - this child proceeded to cry and then say he was really sorry that he lost control. They hugged it out until he felt better, and then he went to school feeling happy, safe, and loved. This is gentle parenting, being there for their emotions and ultimately just not expecting them to behave like adults. This doesn't mean that discipline doesn't exist either, and there will have been times of extreme frustration for the parents (and the child), but being firm can run parallel with being gentle. As I said, gentle parenting is the long game and one day it will just click. When it does, you will have a child who has the ability to process empathy, respect, understanding, and boundaries – skills they will carry with them for their entire lives.

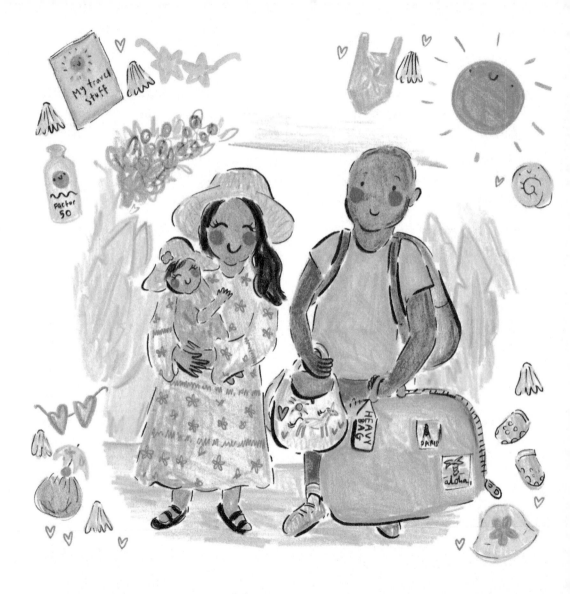

8. Holidays

Ah holidays! Who remembers them? If you are brave enough to be contemplating a holiday with your baby then here's a packing list which might help:

Documents

❏ Passport (Baby/Child passports are only valid for 5 years so make sure your documents are in date!)

Technology

- ❏ Tablet *(with pre downloaded programmes to avoid any wifi issues)*
- ❏ Headphones
- ❏ Phone
- ❏ Chargers
- ❏ Plug Adaptors
- ❏ Baby monitor
- ❏ Night light
- ❏ White noise machine

Clothes

- ❏ Pyjamas/ Sleepsuits
- ❏ Vests
- ❏ Day outfits
- ❏ Sun hats (or winter hats)
- ❏ Swimsuits
- ❏ Socks/tights
- ❏ Shoes
- ❏ Blankets
- ❏ Muslins
- ❏ Sleeping bags

Equipment

- ❏ Pram/Pushchair
- ❏ Pram fan *(if travelling somewhere hot)*
- ❏ Mosquito net for pram
- ❏ Parasol for pram
- ❏ Travel blackout blinds
- ❏ Travel cot
- ❏ Car seat
- ❏ Travel stair gate
- ❏ Cabin suitcase with a baby seat attached (yes, these exist!)

Feeding

- ❑ Formula
- ❑ Bottles
- ❑ Microwave steriliser bags
- ❑ Washing up liquid
- ❑ Bibs
- ❑ Bowls
- ❑ Cutlery
- ❑ Cups
- ❑ Snack boxes
- ❑ So many snacks

Practical Items

- ❑ Medication
- ❑ Paracetamol sachets for hand luggage
- ❑ First Aid kit
- ❑ Bottled water
- ❑ Teethers
- ❑ Dummies
- ❑ Nappies and swim nappies
- ❑ Sling/carrier
- ❑ Toys and teddies
- ❑ Sticker books

Toiletries

- ❑ Hair and body wash
- ❑ Toothbrush/ toothpaste
- ❑ Moisturiser
- ❑ Nappy barrier cream
- ❑ Sunscreen
- ❑ Towels
- ❑ Spare cot bed sheets

After all that, if the list alone hasn't scared you off then don't forget to pack your own bag too!

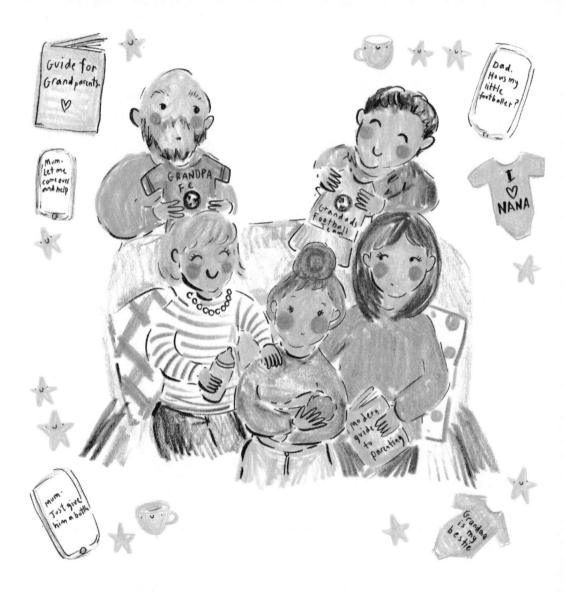

9. In Laws and Other Family Members

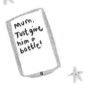

If you're blessed with fantastic in laws and family members, and haven't experienced a single tricky moment since having your baby, then consider yourself really blessed and give yourself permission to skip this chapter and use the time to make a cup of tea or hang the washing that you might have forgotten about (and which has potentially been sat in the washing machine all day since your productive burst this morning - just me?). If on the other hand, you have difficult relationships with family (including in laws) or have great relationships yet have still found certain things a little challenging since having a baby, then this chapter might be useful. Much like becoming a parent, becoming a grandparent doesn't come with a manual.

Grandparents are often excited and can't wait to pass on their experiences. Whilst this comes from a genuine place, what can happen is that it can feel a little interfering especially to a vulnerable new parent. Of course babies are the same now as they've always been, but that doesn't mean that parenting styles haven't evolved or that you might just choose to parent your baby differently. This also doesn't mean that you disapprove of how your parents or in laws parented. See how the awkwardness creeps in? So now that the relationships between your in laws and parents have a new dimension to them, it's time to set some boundaries- it's your child after all. If you don't want your baby to be sat in front of a TV screen/mobile phone/tablet, or you don't want them to be drinking juice, or eating salty and sugary snacks, or taking danger naps which will give you an awful night- then it's absolutely OK to set these rules. What can be hard sometimes, is doing this in a calm and polite way that won't end up coming across rude or leading to offence being taken. My advice here is that it can sometimes help to view the other person's perspective, and tap into how you would take on board the information if you were in their shoes. Perhaps pitching it to them in a way that it's the best thing for the baby, by explaining that your little one could become confused by changing goalposts at home vs at their grandparents house. After all, this is the one thing you hopefully have in common- the mutual contentment of your new family member. These situations are also something that you'll want to be a solid team on with your partner, as it'll be best for them to communicate when it comes to having the conversation with their parents.

If you don't have support from in-laws and/or family members, a little awkwardness is the least of your worries. Hearing from others around you on the childcare support they have for free and on tap can be hard when you don't have the same. Maybe you have parents who would like to help but aren't able to physically or mentally, or you have parents who just don't seem interested, parents who are too busy, you may no longer have your parents, or you could have quite unconventional parental relationships. Whatever it is, it is just really difficult. There's a phrase people often use that raising a child takes a village. Some of us don't have a street let alone a village, and this realisation can be a hard one to swallow. Perhaps you didn't come to this realisation until after you had a child too. So now with the mix of hormones, you find yourself grieving a relationship you thought was there, but in actual fact isn't. Know that it takes time and give yourself permission to allow this time to pass, even over several years. It's normal too, talk to people and you'll be surprised how many others have challenging relationships. On the days when you feel okay to be positive, remind yourself how far you've come. How much you are doing, and how you are a supermum (or dad) for being your child's entire village. Plus, on the bright side, you don't have to deal with that interfering type of in-law or family member who thinks they know best.

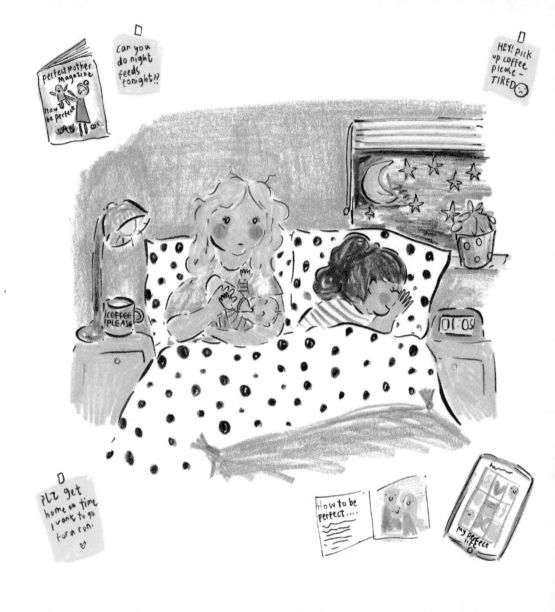

10. Jealousy

When you have a baby one thing is guaranteed, and this is that the dynamic of your relationships will change, from your partner to your friends and family. Let's give the example of the mother as the primary caregiver, and the father whose life doesn't change too much. This can often lead to jealousy or resentment, and so my advice here is to be as supportive to one another as possible. Transitioning from living an independent life, to being a first time mum can be an isolating time for many. Add a partner who is out at work or social events, it is hardly surprising that both jealousy and resentment have the potential to fall into the mix fast. Even when exclusively breastfeeding, it's important for both parents to share their responsibilities as evenly as possible, you're both 50% shareholders. When it comes to household ownership, many couples have blue jobs and pink jobs for example, so perhaps a similar division of labour when it comes to parenthood could also be considered. Give each other time off too, even if it's just to sit in another room within the same house.

It can also help as a mum, to shift your mindset into a different zone to avoid comparing lives with those who don't have the same level of responsibility as you. When you start viewing your role as a full time job, a privilege, or as the person who is lucky enough to (rather than who has to) experience all the firsts, it can really help dispel feelings of negativity. It can also help to know that it is completely normal to feel resentment towards your partner after having a baby. It's okay to acknowledge that feeling and let it be. It is temporary, and it will pass.

When we stop comparing our lives to other people's lives or even to our own past life or imagined future life, it becomes easier to live in a happier present. I hope that little nugget is useful (as a parent or not!)

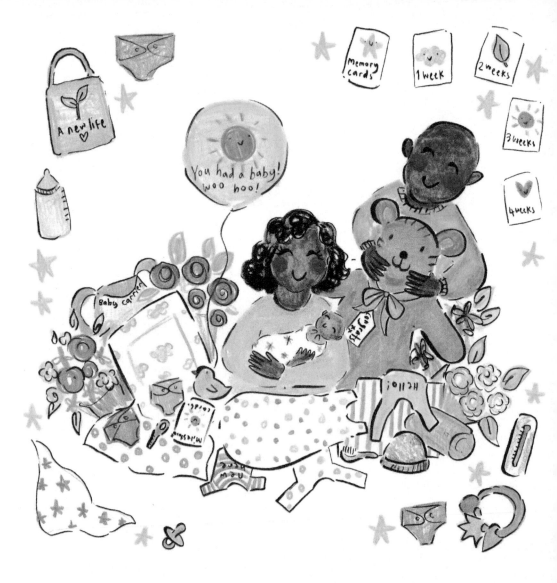

11. Key Items

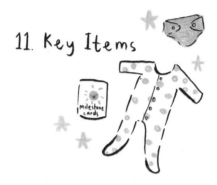

P art of having a new baby is being showered with love, so stock up with vases because there will be lots of flowers! Gifts come in all shapes and sizes, and some are more useful than others. One thing I definitely recommend is having an online gift list. It helps others to know what you would like so that they can get you something genuinely helpful, as well as ensure you receive gifts that aren't duplicated either. With the click of a button, items can be selected and sent to your home address while you're getting everything ready for your little one's arrival. Of course some surprises are still nice, and some people may enjoy shopping for you so the gift list isn't intended to be mandatory by any means. If you do decide to have a gift list, here are some ideas of key items that you may consider adding, with options that cost from £5 to £100 to suit all budgets:

Baby carrier	Baby food maker
Jumperoo	Prep machine
Sleeping bags / swaddles	Play mat
Nappy bin	Car seat mirror
Room thermometer	Waterproof mattress protector
Changing bag / backpack	Night light
Pram suit	Baby light sensory projector
First aid kit	Cot / crib sheets
Bath products	Nail clippers / scissors set
Cellular blankets	Teething toys
Changing mat	Muslins
Moment cards	Top and tail bowl
UV steriliser	Soft hairbrush

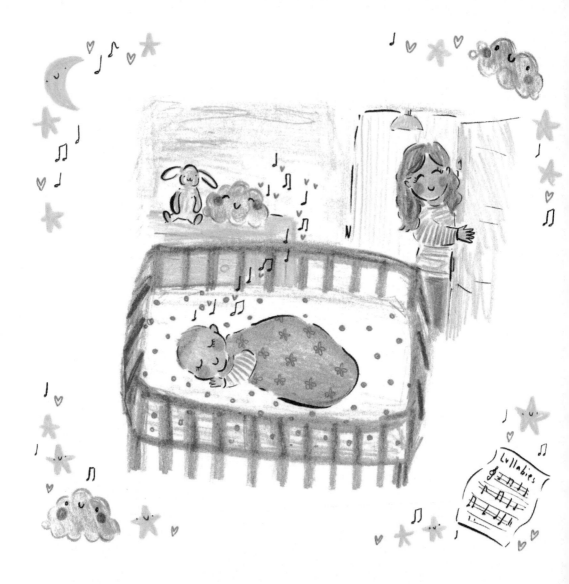

12. Lullabies

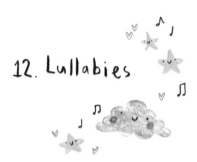

We often hear about white noise for settling babies to sleep. White noise is a crunchy, fairly obnoxious sound resembling an out-of-tune radio station. The bad news is it sounds awful and is enough to give you a headache, but the good news is that there is another option and it's called pink noise. Think along the lines of waves coming into the shore, the sound of gentle rainfall, or a calming lullaby. We often associate lullabies with babies, but I didn't know just how effective they are at helping babies to sleep. It wasn't until Sienna was a few months old that I started obsessing about sleep, as it hadn't been a huge issue until the dreaded sleep regression at around four months. At this time I bought a little device which played a selection of gentle lullabies and had options for various light colours too. There are several of these devices on the market, and it is definitely something I would recommend using. You can control the brightness of the light and volume of the lullaby, as well as various other options from your phone without having the disruption of leaning over to a bedside table. When it comes to babies and sleep, anything is worth a try- right!? Plus being able to tap your phone to pop on the light at the dimmest setting during a night feed is invaluable. Just light enough so you can see what you are doing, but not so light that you risk waking the baby further. From the time I invested in this device, the 'rock a bye baby' lullaby sound was on every night without fail. If I was out and about and needed to get her to sleep, I found it even worked to sing this to her. There are connections with lullabies and the neural pathways in the brain associated with calming and soothing and they can also help with language and cognitive development so it's a win-win. Although it can be recommended to put the lullaby on a timer, so that it's on for long enough to settle your little one without being on for the whole night and potentially becoming a disturbance, I have found that leaving it on all night helped Sienna's sleep. The theory with this is that the sleep environment doesn't change. See what works for your baby, safe in the knowledge that there is no right or wrong and every baby is completely unique and will want what works for them. Whether you have it on part of the time or all night long, opt for pink noise over white noise if like me, you prefer a smoother sound over an amplified audio.

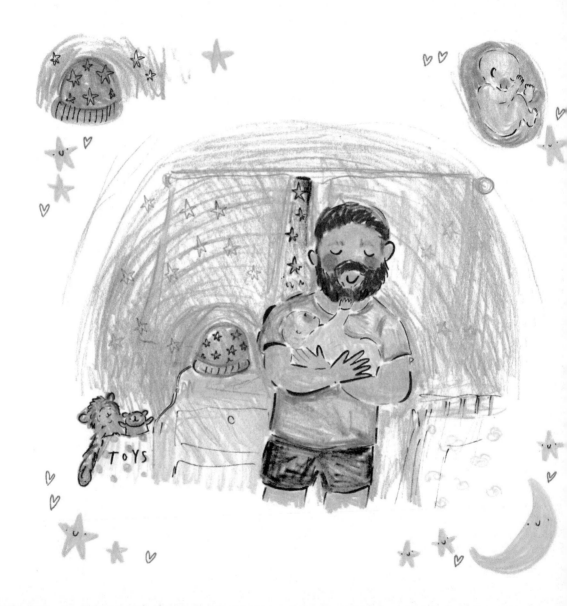

13. Mimicking the Womb

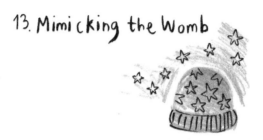

I learnt about mimicking the womb at a local baby class and found it invaluable. It was something new to me that I hadn't heard of before, so I'd like to share it because it can be useful when it comes to comforting your little one, especially during times of need. As well as using this method, I have since read up on the concept and found that it is often referred to as something that can be helpful in the 'fourth' trimester, which is the first 3 months of your baby's life. However there are elements of this that can be used for far longer, so don't be fooled into thinking it's only of short term benefit.

Essentially the idea comes from the simple fact that your baby has been used to being in the womb for 9 months. A safe, warm, comforting environment that one day they were rudely extracted from whether they wanted to be or not. There will be sounds and feelings that they were used to, that you can replicate to help them regain the sense of safe warm comfort that they were once so familiar with.

Generally we might associate this with swaddling, and also with rocking and swaying, but did you also know that gently patting on their bum will be akin to the feeling of your heartbeat against their bum when they were growing inside the womb. So when you are trying to rock your baby to sleep, try a gentle pat on their bum to the same speed as a calm resting pulse to reassure them. We often shush our babies, and the rhythm in which we do this could also mimic the womb to create a more comforting sound. Sometimes we automatically default to a 'shh, shh, shhhhhh' on repeat, but this can be counter productive. In order to mimic the womb, try to make one long continuous shushing sound. This will help to replicate the sound of the blood flowing regularly and smoothly throughout your body, which your baby will have heard as an internal womb noise from the placenta. These two really simple yet really effective tips were invaluable for me in creating a much calmer baby, and I hope you will find them useful too.

I also associate the use of red light with the mimicked womb environment. There are a lot of baby night lights on the market that companies claim will help your baby to sleep using 'red' light, and the explanation which sits alongside this is because it helps to stimulate the body's production of melatonin. I don't dispute this, but I also make the connection here that whilst in the womb, your baby saw light and shape. Although they have blurry vision during their time inside, they can open their eyes from around 27 weeks and respond to bright lights from 31 weeks. During this time the single colour that they see is red. Coincidence? I think not! I'd say that the colour red is therefore able to conjure up the same sense of warmth and comfort as the other tips above, for the reason that it reminds them of their first home.

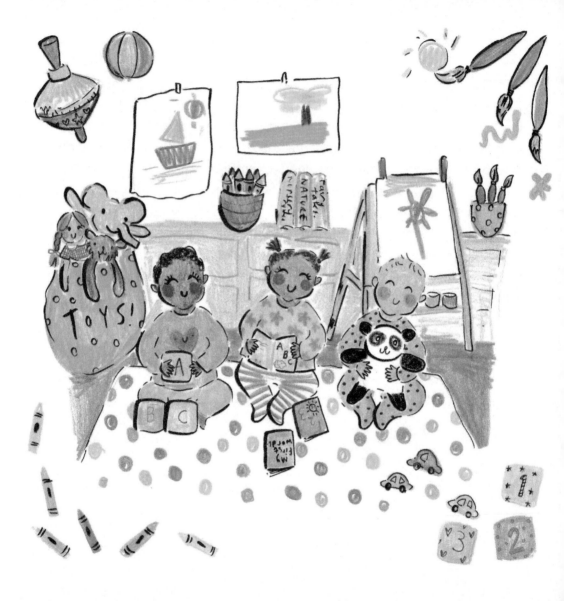

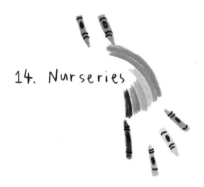

14. Nurseries

Unbeknown to me at the time, it turns out nurseries in some areas have waiting lists of 12+ months. Yes you read that correctly! People put themselves down on waiting lists when they are still pregnant, before their baby has even been born. This isn't just the super duper all singing all dancing nurseries, but pretty much all of them! So consider this chapter a heads up to get researching and organise your post maternity leave childcare, if you plan a return to work.

When looking for a nursery, consider the following checklist and don't be afraid to ask lots of questions to find out the answers. A fellow mum shared a similar list of questions with me when I began looking into nurseries, and although at the time it blew my mind a little bit, these are all things that are very useful to find out. It may help to think of it like an interview, you're the employer as you are quite literally hiring someone to take care of your child. It's the most important recruit you may ever make!

Viewings	Book at least 3 nursery tours. Not just online viewings, but go there in person to physically check them out.
Travel	It's important to factor in your travel time to and from work to help you decide whether you want the nursery to be close to where you work, or where you live.
Costs	Find out whether there are any additional costs besides the daily fee (for food, nappies, milk etc)
Absence	Consider if you still have to pay if your child is not attending for a few days (for instance do sickness charges apply, and do they charge on public holidays?)

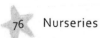

Payments	How are fees paid? Is it monthly in advance, for example. Do they accept payments from the government's childcare tax free account? Check this out if you haven't, it's a great scheme to help pay for your childcare - currently set at a £2 top up for every £8 you pay in. You can only apply 1 month before the child starts nursery, so bear this in mind and check if your prospective nursery will accept the payment scheme.
Opening times	Are drop off and collection times flexible? Some nurseries charge late collection fees so find out if this might apply.
Behaviour	Find out what their behaviour policy is and consider if you agree with it (such as use of the naughty step and how they might respond if a child bites for example).
Outdoor Space	Do they have a garden, and are the children allowed to use this area everyday? Is it suitable for all weather? If not, how would you feel about your child being in one room all day from drop off to collection?

Food	Do they provide food, and if so is it cooked onsite? Ask for a sample menu. Ask to see their food hygiene certificate. If they don't provide food, are you expected to provide a packed lunch? Consider the time implications this will have for your morning routine.
Staffing Ratios	During your visit, try to notice if the staffing ratios are appropriate in each room. It's a legal requirement for there to be a minimum of 1 member of staff for every 3 babies (under 2 years) and 1 member of staff for every 4 children/toddlers (over age 2).
Qualifications	What are the qualifications of all staff? The bare minimum is Level 2, but consider if this is enough for you, or perhaps you would like to find a nursery where the staff have Level 3 or above. Ask to see the manager's qualification, and although not a legal requirement ideally this should be a Level 6.
First Aid	Are all staff qualified in First Aid? Legally only 1 person in the building is required to be, but perhaps you would like to find a nursery that exceeds this base level requirement. Do they have an accident policy or record? Can you ask to see the book?

Staff	What is their staff turnover? (Settings with a high staff turnover may indicate an issue, or point towards instability in who will be caring for your child). Are the staff diverse, or are they all the same demographic? Consider if this is an issue to you.
Medicine Policy	Can your child attend when on medication? Are the staff able to administer the medication?
Screen Time	Do they have / use TV? If so, for how long? Consider if you would be happy paying for your child to be sat in front of a screen for long periods.
Settling In	How do settling-in sessions work? Are you allowed to stay with your child for the first day or first week? Or are you expected to drop and go.
Special Education Needs	If applicable, will your child be allocated a key worker?
Feedback	How often will you receive feedback on your child's progression? Do they share completed paperwork with you, and what will this look like?

Curriculum	Nurseries have a curriculum, you should be able to download this so you have something useful to follow and use when assessing your child's milestones.
Nappies	What is their nappy changing policy? For instance is there a key person who will change your child's nappy, or do all staff change babies nappies? Do the nursery provide the nappies or are you expected to leave a nappy bag?
Environment	Although it's important to look at the resources when you view the nursery, also take time to assess the child relationships. It's one thing to have a top of the range building with plenty of toys and great facilities, but if the staff aren't great with the children then it's not going to benefit your child as much as an old building with limited resources but highly skilled staff who are completely engaged with your child. The latter will result in far greater positive outcomes for children.

Ofsted	Remember to read the most recent Ofsted report which will be published online. Consider how recent it was last evaluated too.
Safeguarding	Ask what their safeguarding policy is and if you could see a copy of it.
Security	Do they operate a password system for you to send someone else to pick up your child? Can children get out (or strangers in) easily, or are there measures in place to prevent this?
Routine	What is the routine of the day? Are all children expected to sleep at the same time? Is it free play or do they have structured activities?

As you can see, there are a lot of things to consider but you won't need to necessarily ask it all in one go. Generally, you'll get a feel for the right nursery fairly early on and can then gradually find out the rest.

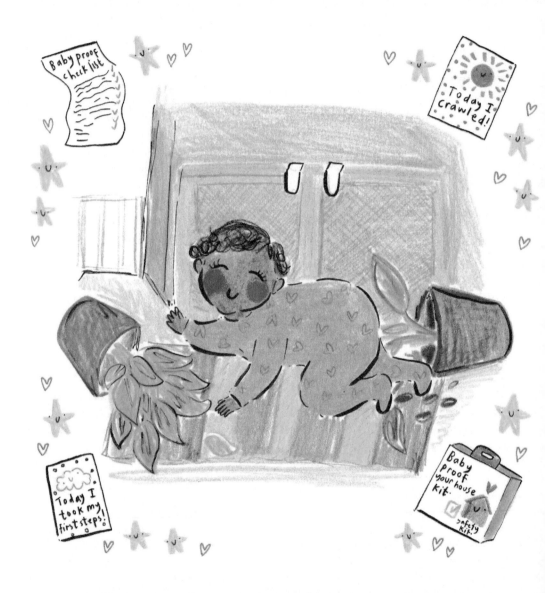

15. On the Move

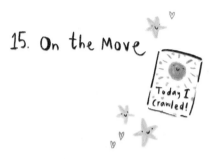

Today I Crawled!

In the blink of an eye your baby, who was once laying gently on his or her back kicking their legs on a playmat and grasping for hanging toys within reach, will be on the move! There are some things you can do to help prepare your baby for this exciting development, for instance tummy time is great for building strength in your little ones muscles. Did you know, a cuddle with your baby lying on your chest even counts as tummy time until they feel comfortable to do this on a mat. Just a few seconds every now and again to begin with is more than enough too, think little and often.

When they take their first crawl it's so exciting, and it's at this point that things start to get interesting. Before you know it they'll be into everything, that's how they learn after all. I found that this is when baby proofing the house from a safety point of view became really important. This next bit might be a little scary to read but it's good to know that the following risk factors are very real and result in tens of thousands of accidents every year with little ones. Bringing your awareness to these risks is not intended to scare you, but instead to focus your attention on some considerations to help keep your little one safe and sound.

Category	Risk
Choking	If it's small enough to fit in their mouth- keep it out of reach. Examples include **buttons, coins, small toy parts** (especially prevalent in toys designed for older children), even **fluff/yarn** from a woolly jumper, and anything which includes **batteries**. In particular, the small silver button batteries are very dangerous. These are not only a choking hazard but they cause severe internal burns if swallowed and can lead to death.

Category	Risk
Suffocation	More things to keep out of reach to reduce this risk. These include **carrier bags**, and **nappy bags**. If you have a nappy bin in the nursery and tend to overlap the bag around the rim of the lid, keep it away from your baby's cot where they could reach and put it in their mouth. As well as plastic bags, consider the risk of **bed sheets** and **covers/throws** which your little one could reach and pull down from a bed or sofa causing entrapment.
Strangulation	Another risk mitigated by keeping things out of reach, yes it's a theme that runs throughout this table! This one includes **curtain and blind cords**- these can quickly wrap around a baby or toddler's neck, but can so easily be tied up out of reach to stop this happening. Also don't leave any **dressing gown cords** or **drawstring bags** lying around- all rope or cord must be out of reach for obvious reasons. Then there is the risk associated with **bannisters or balcony railings**- often the gaps between the rails are more than 2.5 inches which means small babies can fit their bodies through, before getting stuck around their neck/head area. Cover these areas with safety netting.

Category	Risk
Poisoning	**Medicines, cleaning products** and **laundry/dishwasher** capsules should all be locked away or stored in a cupboard high enough so they are out of reach and sight. Some cleaning products contain a bittering agent designed to make it taste awful enough to reduce the chances of children swallowing them, so opt for these when shopping. **E-cigarettes and their refills** should also be kept out of reach because the nicotine is poisonous and very dangerous for little ones. Also consider if any **plants** in your garden could be poisonous.
Glass related injury	If any of your **internal doors** have glass at a low enough level, make sure it's safety glass which won't shatter so easily. If you have a **greenhouse**, consider fencing this off or installing safety glazing. Never let your baby within reach of anything that is made of glass. If something like a **glass tumbler** does get broken, then dispose of it quickly and safely- wrapping it up in newspaper for example before it goes into the bin.

Category	Risk
Burns/Scalds	**Hot drinks** should be kept away from all young children, even 15 minutes after being made it could cause a scald to their gentle skin so don't risk it. Mugs can look fun with the bright colours, so out of sight is best to avoid any temptation for little hands to try and reach. The **kettle** can also be grabbed and pulled down if the wire is hanging loose, so keep any cords short and out of reach. When cooking, use the rings at the back of **the hob** and face the saucepan handles to the back so they can't be grabbed or knocked by accident. Other risk factors include **hair straighteners and curling irons, matches and lighters, button batteries and laundry capsules** which can cause internal burns. Overall, keep them all out of reach.
Drowning	Ensure any **garden ponds** that your baby has access to are fenced off or covered securely. If you're using a **paddling pool,** empty it as soon as you've finished. Never leave your baby unattended in the **bath.**

Category	Risk
Fires	If you have a **fireplace,** always keep it completely enclosed using a fireguard that attaches to the wall and don't hang or place anything on the guard. Keep any **matches** and **lighters** away from reach.

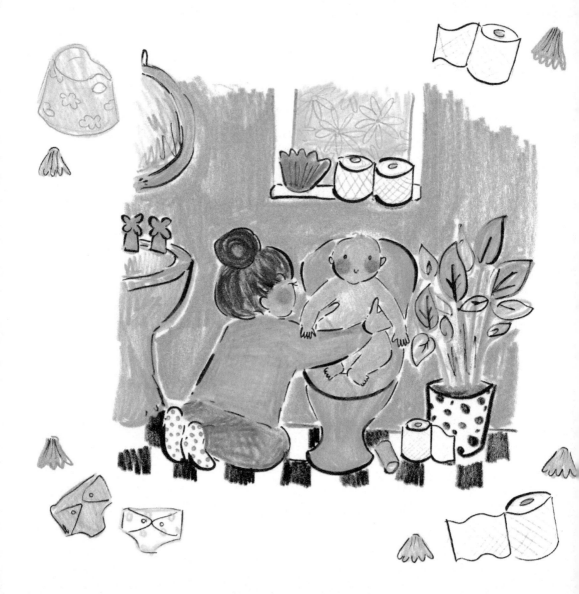

16. Potty Training

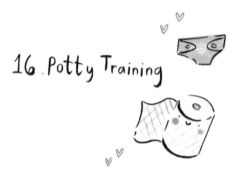

raditionally, potty training takes place any time from around 18-24 months, and sometimes not until 3 years of age. However, there is a school of thought about 'infant' potty training which would suggest it's easier to start younger, since an older child will have to not only learn the new behaviour but will also have to unlearn what they've been doing their whole life up until now. Infant potty training can start anywhere from birth to 4 months and essentially works by anticipation. By this I mean that it's a case of anticipating when your baby is going to relieve themselves and then rushing them to the nearest bathroom. According to this theory, your baby will be completely toilet trained by around the 18 month mark.

Personally, I had no idea how to detect if Sienna was going to the toilet in her nappy. She has obviously always been quite good at multitasking, or just carrying on her 'business' as usual in both senses of the word. If you're reading this and thinking the same, then I'd just encourage you to look less at the finish line and more at the track. What do I mean by this? Okay, so have you ever been mid-nappy change and your baby has peed all over you, and the changing mat/table? Perhaps this is in fact what we have 'trained' them to do all along, without knowing it. When changing your baby's nappy next time, consider taking them to the bathroom and holding them in a seated position over the toilet when you remove the nappy. Hold them there for a few moments to give them the opportunity to go. This essentially might start 'training' your baby to make an association between going to the toilet in this environment and position, rather than in their nappy whilst lying down on a mat. Of course this might not result in the ability to stop using nappies as soon as infant training might advertise, let alone be able to detect when your baby will need to go, but you'll be encouraging your baby to start practising a skill that will most certainly be used later on, which when you look at it like this, what have you got to lose?!

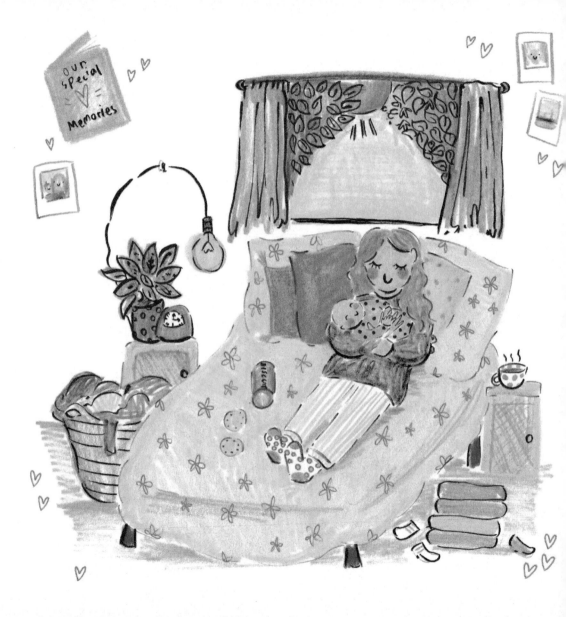

17. Quality Time

Time, it's the one thing we all want more of. Without being morbid, it's a fact that the only guarantee in life is death. Gosh that's depressing isn't it? Let's flip the script and focus on what we can control. I remember being about 10 years old and having the great fortune of being in Malaysia with my family. We were visiting a tea plantation in the Cameron Highlands when I found interest in a small handmade jewellery stall. I was lucky and was bought a necklace with a Malay scribe which I was told read 'you can live life, or exist life'. This quote has stayed with me ever since and so when I find myself floating along in my comfort zone I think back to this and give myself a little nudge. One day when we are at the end of our lives, it's the quality time we have spent making memories that I imagine we will look back on with a smile. Of course we have to work, and there will always be an endless cycle of jobs around the house but this chapter is a reminder to spend time living in the moment, the only time that really exists. Spend quality time with your baby and never feel guilty for it.

Those first few days, weeks and months of having a newborn baby are precious and as such are often referred to as the honeymoon phase. Soak it up, stay in bed all day in your pyjamas and cuddle as much as you can. Don't rush to get out and show off your baby or have people over to the house, they can wait. This is your time to recover, to bask in the glory of the little human you have created, and to bond. While you may feel that you are not achieving much, remind yourself of how important this time is for developing a sense of security for your baby. I say this because sometimes as parents we struggle to be selfish and prioritise our needs so if you won't do it for yourself, do it for your baby. Quality time with your baby might include skin to skin to regulate their breathing and heart rate, giving them a massage, making eye contact during a feed, responding to every cry to help your baby build trust in you, kissing your baby while they still let you (they'll grow up fast and find you embarrassing at some point), smiling, singing, reading, and cuddling. Now this is a to-do list worth getting behind! These are all ways to aid in the development of bonding and attachment, and they make for the best memories. So put your phone away and put a hold on any plans, people will understand that you may take several hours or days to reply. These cuddles won't be here forever.

It is also important to make quality time for yourself during this time. It may be important, but let's be honest it can also be extremely challenging to do this. You might not even want to be away from your baby (see chapter 4 on primary maternal preoccupation). So during the newborn phase in particular, it might be helpful to re-shift your thinking when it comes to the definition of quality time. For now, think small snippets of 'you' time: a shower, a cup of tea, or even a bath while your little one is in the bouncer next to you. You don't have to be far from your baby to enjoy a moment of time for yourself. Perhaps some yoga practice at home with your baby (see chapter 25 for more on yoga), or a walk in nature with your baby in the pram while you get some fresh air and listen to a podcast or a favourite soundtrack as you walk. These small moments of relief could make a big impact on your mental health.

Lastly, this is your reminder to make quality time for your partner. If you have limited support and aren't able to go out together, it's still possible to spend some quality time at home. Even if your baby doesn't sleep for long stretches,

I'd encourage you to grab 10 minutes to focus on each other. Postpone the urge to collapse in a heap or submerge into screen time. A game of scrabble on the sofa can be a nice way to tune out of the days which can sometimes feel monotonous, and be present. Failing that, why wait for an evening? Make weekends fun and book some day trips, see chapter 24 for some useful tips on making this as easy as possible. Whatever you do, do it for you. For yourself, your partner, and your baby. Put the people pleasing to the bottom of your priority list and make some guilt free happy memories as a family. 'I really regret spending quality time', said no one, ever.

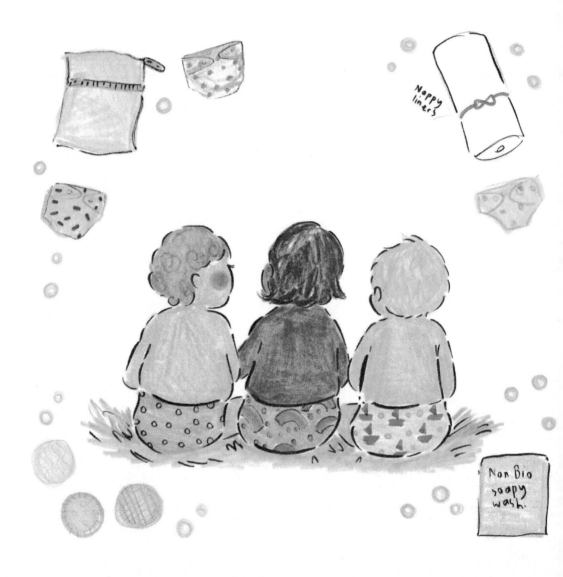

18. Reusables

There can be a lot of wastage with babies, but there are options to reduce your newly increased impact on the environment. Of course when you're getting your head around being a parent there is often enough to do without adding to the equation, so this chapter is by no means intended to overwhelm you. Plus you don't have to decide straight away- a switch to reusables when your little one is 6 months old will still have a huge benefit on the environment, and even a partial switch helps. If we consider nappies alone, the environmental impact is scary! In the UK for instance, there's something like 8 million nappies disposed of every single day and each one takes 500 years to degrade in a landfill. To know that the nappies you and I would have worn as babies are still hanging around on the planet was enough to shock me into trying reusables! Once I did, I was surprised how easy it is. The business case stacks up too, since buying reusables is an investment which soon pays for itself in the money you'd be endlessly spending on disposables.

You can buy 'birth to potty' reusable nappies, which means not worrying about what size to get for your growing baby as these nappies adjust via velcro or poppers depending on the style and brand you opt for. I found the velcro ones easiest, and the most similar to disposables in terms of how simple they are to put on.

Top Tip: Make sure you stick the velcro tabs together before putting them in the wash, which prevents them from losing the stick.

You can also get a 'wet bag', to keep in your changing bag. This is ideal for popping in a dirty reusable nappy or liner until you get home.

The most complicated thing I found to get my head around, was the difference between 'boosters' and 'liners', as well as the purpose of these. The booster tucks into a little pocket in the back of the nappy to add extra absorbency, whereas the liner goes between the nappy and your baby's bum to catch the contents! The best liners in my opinion are the fleecy ones, which are so luxuriously soft that it makes the disposable nappies seem like wearing a newspaper. You can preload the nappies, so that the boosters and liners are in place and ready to go for when you need them, and some nappies even have built in boosters. When it comes to changing time, you don't always need a new nappy either, you can often just change the inserts for new ones. If it's a poo you'll need to change the whole thing though, because quite often the poo won't land neatly on the liner- that would be far too easy!

Then there's the washing requirement. This is where it's simply about getting a rhythm of having a load dry and stuffed ready for a changing bag whilst another set is drying, and as the bucket fills washing a load whilst stuffing the ones that have dried in the meantime, so that you can restock the cupboard. I'd say a safe bet is to invest in about 30 nappies so there could be 10 dirty, 10 drying and 10 in use, with the cycle constantly moving. In terms of the bucket, you can get ones with lids and liner bags that keep the odour locked whilst making it easy to grab the bag and put it in the machine without touching anything gross.

> **Top Tip**: A useful tip is to run them through on a rinse cycle before your usual cycle, with the addition of a natural washing powder.

If you're thinking of giving it a go, here's a useful shopping list based on the above, which you can of course adapt to suit you:

- ❏   30 birth to potty (BTP) velcro nappies with built in boosters
- ❏   30 fleecy liners
- ❏   1 wet bag
- ❏   1 nappy bin
- ❏   1 pot of natural washing powder

Nappies aren't the only reusable opportunity, as once you've got the hang of these you could expand to reusable wipes instead of baby wipes, which like the nappies are much softer for your little ones bum. Similarly, it takes a little getting used to but once you've set up the logistics around washing it's easy.

Reusable toys exist too. There are toy subscription services out there, which aren't just sustainable but make sense for you to avoid having old toys lying around. You can keep a constant turnover of interesting toys for your little learner whilst helping to reduce your impact on the environment and save spending on new ones. Or on a smaller level, you could set something similar up with friends who have babies of a similar age. Check out local charity shops too to keep the circular economy going.

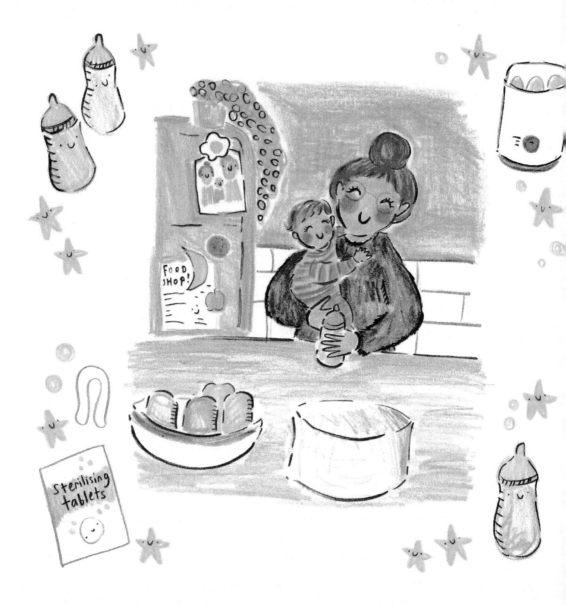

19. Sterilising

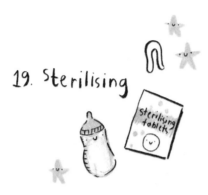

abies have immune systems which aren't fully developed and so it's very important to sterilise their feeding equipment. Even if you're planning to breastfeed it's good to learn the importance of sterilising because at some point you may wish to introduce a bottle, or you might find breastfeeding doesn't work out for you.

When Sienna and I were in the hospital for the first 5 days of her life, and my milk was delayed due to the blood I lost in labour, I bottle fed her to prevent her weight loss plummeting below 10%. This was something I found myself completely unprepared for. The hospital provided me with bottles and my husband dropped off some ready made formula milk. A midwife then showed me that by boiling a kettle and pouring the water into a large jug, I could hold the bottle of milk in that jug of hot water to prepare the bottle. What I didn't know is that the bottle and teat they had provided were 'pre-sterilised', and that this preparation was just bringing the milk to a nice drinking temperature but not actually sterilising the bottle. Fast forward a day or so later, I was told by another midwife that I wasn't entitled to anymore of the hospital bottles and should by now be providing my own. I didn't have any but with next day delivery at my fingertips, I was able to order some for my husband to bring to the hospital. I continued the preparation I'd been taught, but Sienna would be sick and the midwives would tell me this was normal. However, mothers instinct kicked in and I knew something wasn't right. It wasn't until a kinder midwife told me about sterilising bags that I was horrified to find I hadn't been sterilising her bottles correctly. To this day, I'm still upset by this. As a first time mum in the hospital completely alone, recovering from a traumatic labour, and with no support- it's fair to say I was in a bit of a daze. Ever since this day I've made it my mission to learn and know everything there is to know about looking after my daughter. It sounds silly now, but all the preparation I had done in the lead up to her birth involved either preparing for the labour or preparing for physical items that she needed at home. So with wishing someone explained the following to me, here I am now sharing it with you.

You can sterilise via a number of different techniques. Here are some options:

Cold Water

This method uses a dissolvable tablet in water, which creates a sterilising solution that you need to submerge items in for at least 30 minutes.

Steam

There are different types of steam sterilisers on the market, some plug into the mains and some can be used in conjunction with your microwave. You can also use reusable microwave sterilising bags which you add the items to with some water in the bottom of the bag, and pop in the microwave. These are really handy when you're on the go, or in the hospital and have limited equipment or space available.

UV

Much like the steam sterilisers, these are units that you can purchase. However, unlike steam they don't use any heat so you don't need to worry about cooling items down before use, and they sterilise in around 3 minutes with little to no hassle.

Boiling Water

This method involves submerging the items in boiling water for at least 10 minutes.

For the first 12 months of your baby's life, sterilise all feeding equipment every single time you use it. As soon as you've used bottles, breast-pumps, teats or any other milk storage / collection / feeding equipment, wash them with warm soapy water. You can opt to use a dishwasher for this part for most items. Once you've washed them, use cold running water to rinse it all, and then they are ready to be sterilised again.

This is one of those things that sounds more complicated than it is. Once you know how you're going to do it, and have done it once or twice, it becomes second nature.

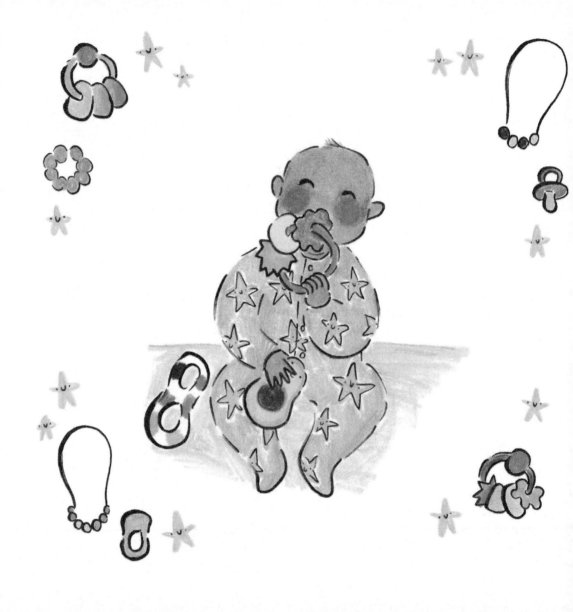

20. Teething

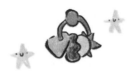

A painful topic for many in more ways than one, teething often gets a bad name and so can be blamed for everything. A bad night's sleep, must be teething! Your baby is not eating well, teething! Explosive nappies, you guessed it, teething! The list goes on. Of course, there are genuine symptoms to look out for when it comes to teething but it isn't always the case that when your baby seems a little out of character, that teething must be to blame. That said, it is also useful to know that your little one can be teething without any teeth actually coming through. This is because their teeth move up through their gums before breaking the surface. During this phase of movement your baby can be in real pain, and quite often it's this 'pre-teething' stage that lasts the longest. Think of it like laying the foundations for a building, this is when all the hard work goes in without anything yet to show for it. Your poor baby has all the pain, and no gain! Then all of a sudden the building starts to take shape, and the interior design comes together in a flash. How long this process takes depends on several factors, and the same applies to teething. Your baby could start teething when they are just a few months old, or maybe much later. Either way it's fairly safe to say that by their 1st birthday you will more than likely have a baby with teeth, or a tooth coming soon!

Generally speaking, teething symptoms could look like one or more of the following:

 Red gums, which are also sore so your baby may show signs of irritation
 A high temperature
 Rosy cheek(s)
 Excessive dribble
 Paying more attention to their mouth- for instance they may pout their lips or blow bubbles
 Pulling their ear(s)- also a sign of tiredness just to confuse you
 Chewing on anything and everything
 Sleep regressions

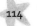

It is always horrible for us and our babies when they are in pain, so of course we want to do everything we can to mitigate this for them as much as possible. My advice is to get yourself a variety of teething rings and toys, make sure they are sterilised (see chapter 19), and keep them in the fridge because the cold temperature can help to soothe your baby's gums. When taking a sterilised teether out and about with you, a zip lock bag is useful to keep it safe from germs. If your baby is over 6 months and onto the weaning phase (see chapter 23), things like carrot sticks and other healthy fruits and vegetables can be helpful for them to chew on and relieve pain. You can also gently massage their gums with a clean finger to offer some light relief. If all else fails, distraction is a great tactic, playtime is always a winner! When it comes to medicating for the pain associated with teething, there are gels and powders that might be useful- though bear in mind there has been limited research carried out on the effectiveness of these. Lastly, if your little one has a high temperature then paracetamol or ibuprofen will be helpful at this stage, with ibuprofen the more effective of these two options when it comes to teething due to its anti inflammatory impacts.

When their teeth do start coming through, you may notice the bottom front teeth making an appearance first (incisors), then the top two incisors, before the two either side of the top (lateral incisors), then the bottom two lateral incisors. Generally speaking, once these are through you'll start to see the first molars around 12-16 months followed by the canines which are in between the lateral incisors and the molars, and then finally their second molars. As the teeth start breaking through the gums, it's good to start brushing them which you can do using a tiny smear of fluoride toothpaste to begin with. Doing this is not only beneficial for their dental hygiene but also helps to bring this into a habitual routine for your baby to get used to. It is advised that you stop using a dummy if you have been doing so, ideally when your baby is around 12 months but definitely in line with their teeth breaking through. This is because the teeth can actually move to make space for the dummy, creating what's called an 'open bite'.

All in all, their full set of around 20 teeth should be through by the time your little one is 30 months. So it's a long hard slog from when your baby is just a few months old to almost 3 years of age during which they will have been teething on and off. Some babies are more affected than others when it comes to teething, so just take it as it comes and try not to stress too much.

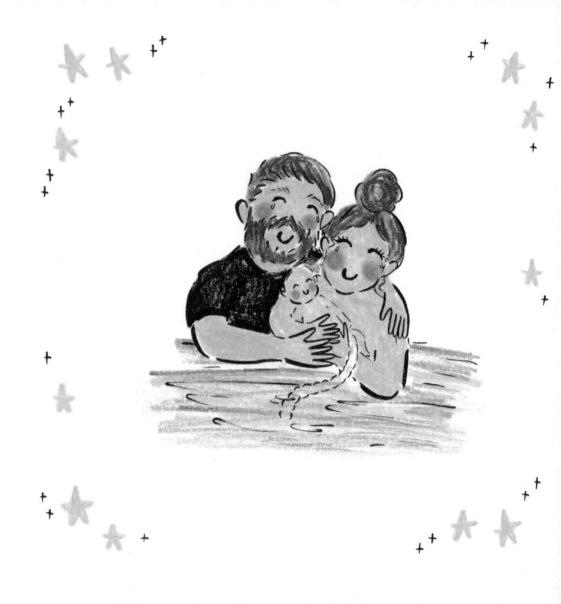

21. Umbilical Cord

This chapter is for the pre and post birth considerations specifically relating to the umbilical cord. It's a short but important one (the chapter too). Let's start with the pre birth bit. When you find yourself writing your birth plan or preferences, consider what you would like to happen to the umbilical cord. Not sure why it's something key to consider? The umbilical cord has been the supply to your baby since you were about 5 weeks pregnant, delivering both nutrients and oxygen. When your baby is born you have some options to consider for the cord and since you may not be in a decision making state, advanced consideration is helpful here.

Delayed cord clamping. This equates to anything longer than 1 minute (usually no more than 5) and is generally normal practice these days. Guidelines state that it is better for your baby if you wait until the cord has stopped pulsating and turned white before you cut the cord. Even though it's fairly standard procedure, you should still specify whether this is your preference or not on your birth plan. If there are any complications with the delivery, such as breathing difficulties with your baby, then the cord will likely be clamped sooner. It's important to know this, since it was a shock to me when Sienna's cord was clamped much closer to the 1 minute than 5. Whilst the consultant assured me this was still 'delayed', I wasn't convinced at the time. However, looking back with the knowledge I have now, this will have been due to the complications in labour as they were concerned for Sienna's wellbeing having been unable to identify her little heartbeat. Knowledge is power as they say, so I hope this information helps you to worry less, should you find yourself in a similar situation.

Blood donation. I have to admit I didn't know anything about this when I was pregnant but have since read up on it and wanted to include it in this chapter so, if like me you don't know much about this option, you will have some information to consider. By donating the umbilical cord after birth, the stem cells in the cord blood can be used for a stem cell transplant and so your baby could potentially be a lifesaver from day one! The placenta is normally thrown away with the cord blood in it, however if you opt to donate the blood you won't notice much difference other than the midwife asking for verbal or written consent to proceed with the donation. The donation is then taken care of independently so it won't take the midwife's attention away from you or your baby. As well as this, the blood isn't collected from the placenta until after the baby is born, after the cord is cut (including if you've delayed the cord clamping) and after the placenta has been delivered, so it poses no risk to you or your baby.

Either way your little one will be left with a stump, and a small plastic clamp on top. This usually falls off naturally around 1-3 weeks after the birth (don't be tempted to pull it off, even if it is only hanging by a thread). Until it falls off you need to keep it dry as this speeds up the healing process, and by keeping it clean and dry you are also helping to prevent infection. Bathing your baby via a top and tail method will help with keeping the cord dry (see chapter 2 on bathing for more on how to do this), as will folding the front of the nappy down so that it doesn't cover the cord. A lot of nappies have a section that makes doing this quite easy. Other than this, it is best to leave it alone really! If you notice any swelling, redness, or odours coming from the cord do contact your health visitor or GP as these can be signs of infection.

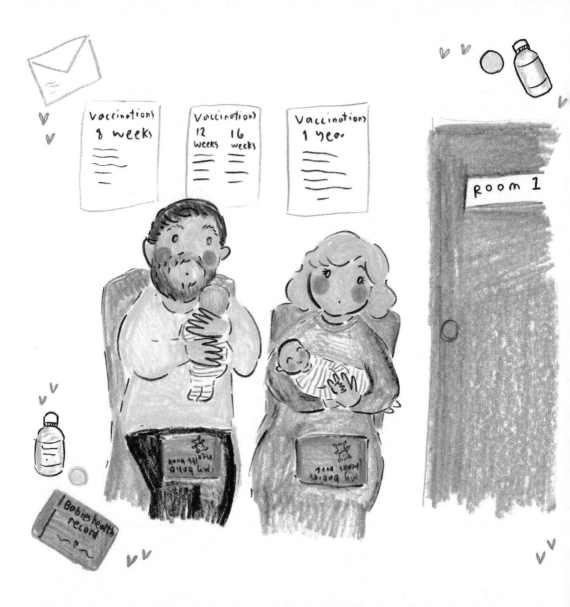

22. Vaccinations

Your brand new baby is born and you feel ready to show him or her off to the world! Be mindful of the fact that your baby will have a very immature immune system, so it may be wise to wait until some of the vaccinations have been given before going too crazy. This chapter isn't designed to advise you in any way around what to do, but is instead intended to give you a heads up on what vaccinations your little one will be entitled to, at what intervals, and thus what appointments you should expect to start making with your local GP practice once your little baby is here.

The following summary covers the 4 sets of vaccination appointments you'll need within the first year of your baby's life:

Age	Vaccinations	Protection against
8 weeks	2 injections (one in each thigh) and 1 set of drops in the mouth.	Diphtheria Tetanus Pertussis (whooping cough) Polio Haemophilus influenzae type b (Hib) Hepatitis B Rotavirus Meningococcal group B disease (MenB)
12 weeks	2 injections (one in each thigh) and 1 set of drops in the mouth.	Diphtheria Tetanus Pertussis (whooping cough) Polio, Hib Hepatitis B Pneumococcal disease Rotavirus

Age	Vaccinations	Protection against
16 weeks	2 injections (one in each thigh).	Diphtheria Tetanus Pertussis (whooping cough) *polio Hib Hepatitis B MenB
1 year	4 injections (two in each thigh).	Hib/Meningococcal group C (MenC) MenB Measles, mumps, rubella (MMR) Pneumococcal disease

The side effects vary with each baby, although as you've gathered by now, everything varies with each baby. I found that Sienna was a little upset and clingy after each round of vaccinations. As per our GP's advice, we gave Sienna some paracetamol straight after the vaccinations. This is generally recommended to prevent a high temperature, rather than waiting for it to come and acting reactively and this worked for us. I have heard of side effects being more severe, with some leading to sickness and interrupting sleep as a result so bear that in mind too. In terms of general preparedness, you may find it easiest to dress your baby in a sleepsuit for the vaccination appointments. This means not having to get them undressed, as you can just undo the poppers to get their legs out, which just makes everything a little simpler for you whilst being more comfortable for your little one. Although Sienna was a summer baby, I imagine this to be even more useful in the winter to avoid your baby getting cold as well as having to face the needles. Overall, the appointments are very quick and although your baby will cry, they will usually stop crying before you've even left the room.

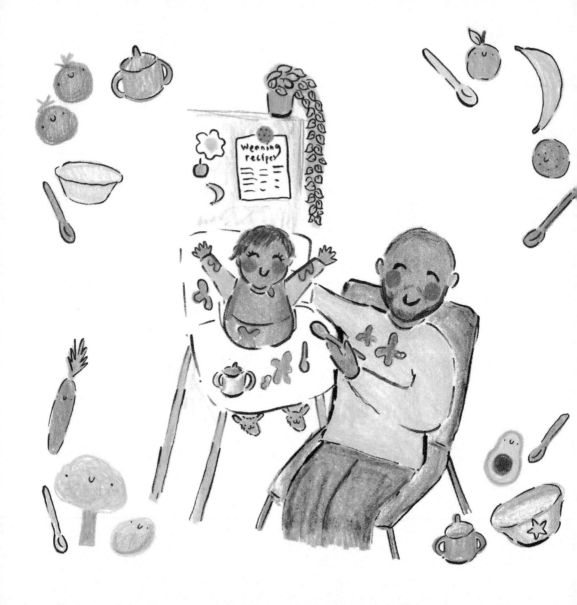

23. Weaning

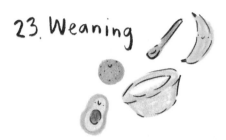

Weaning, this is when you look back at the newborn phase and think how 'easy' it seems in comparison. Of course, at the time it was far from easy because it was so new to you and you were learning everything about that phase. Now we move onto learning everything about weaning. From the foods you can and can't offer, to the choking fear, and a sample menu, I'm hoping this chapter gives you the tools and guidance you need to help weaning seem a little easier. After all, by this time you will have accomplished so much already that you can do this and soon enough it'll be a doddle too.

The ABC's of weaning.

A- Let's start with allergens. It's important to establish if your baby has any allergies, so ensure to introduce allergens gradually. The general rule of thumb is to introduce allergens 3 days apart because reactions can be delayed.

B- Always have a beaker of water on the high chair. Ideally a 'free flowing' cup, as per dentist recommendations. At 6 months they can have water that doesn't have to be boiled, though you might like to filter it.

C- When it comes to choking, this is a valid fear factor for us all. There are some things you can do to help reduce the risk. Chop foods into small pieces, avoiding disc shapes when chopping foods like carrots, bananas, sausages etc. You'll spend a lot of time sat on the edge of your seat holding your breath in fear of your baby choking. It's a normal fear though is often confused with gagging, which is still not nice. My advice is to do a baby first aid course to prepare yourself for every eventuality because whilst there are things we can do to prevent choking, it does unfortunately happen.

S- Be very wary of salt, their little kidneys are too immature to handle any more than 1 gram of salt per day. You can buy things like low/no salt stock cubes and low salt butter to help reduce the salt content where possible. Remember that there are hidden salts in bread and cheese as well as in processed meats like ham. We often add these foods as part of wider recipes, so just be aware of these hidden salts to ensure babies aren't exceeding the recommended amount.

When you first start weaning, usually around 6 months, my advice is to offer some puree with a side of finger food for 'play'. You can get bowls with different sections that make it quite easy to put this out on one plate. A puree in the middle section, with the finger foods at the side usually works well. Why not just puree? Of course that's OK if it is more convenient for you, but eating is a complicated set of tasks that your baby needs to learn. From seeing the food, to picking it up, finding their mouth, putting it in, and learning how to manipulate it in their mouth to break it down for chewing, it's a lot! Babies are born with the ability to swallow, but chewing is a learnt process.

Once you've tested for allergens and your baby is confident picking food up and putting it to their mouth, you'll find they probably grow out of the puree stage quite naturally. This is where it gets a little easier because you can make family meals to suit the baby too. You'll find that your baby eats more on some days than others, they may love banana porridge on some days and hate it on others. Try not to worry too much about this, remembering the phrase 'under one is just for fun' helped me with this. It's all about learning and experiencing different tastes and textures.

If you start weaning at 6 months with breakfast, you could consider adding dinners at 7 months, and then lunches from 8 or 9 months as an example. Here's a sample menu that I used from around 8.5 months for Sienna to eat, throw on the floor, play with, wipe up the walls...you know the drill:

	Breakfast	Lunch	Dinner
Monday	Porridge Blended oats with a choice of fruit.	Eggs Boiled, scrambled.	Pasta With sauces such as butternut squash and tomato, creamy mushroom, or cream cheese and courgette.
Tuesday	Weetabix Softened in the microwave, with choice of fruit.	Jacket Potato Fillings such as tuna, cheese and chive, or vegetables.	Chicken Endless options such as lemon chicken strips with asparagus, chicken stir fry, chicken fajitas, chicken casserole.
Wednesday	Yoghurt Greek yoghurt with choice of fruit.	Pinwheels Fillings such as pesto, cheese, spinach, or tomato.	Mince Spaghetti bolognaise, shepherds pie, lasagne, or burgers.

	Breakfast	Lunch	Dinner
Thursday	**Porridge** Blended oats with a choice of fruit.	**Toast** Spreads such as avocado, peanut butter, hummus, or mashed banana.	**Veg** Cauliflower cheese, broccoli and potato bake.
Friday	**Weetabix** Softened in the microwave, with choice of fruit.	**Muffin Pots** Crustless mini quiche / egg muffins with fillings such as spinach, tomato, or cheese.	**Fish** Cod with sweet potato, salmon and pea risotto, or tuna fish pie.
Saturday	**Waffles** Served with a choice of fruit topping.	**Fritters** With fillings such as vegetables, peas, sweetcorn, bananas, or blueberries.	**Curry** Lentil, chickpea, vegetable, spinach etc.

	Breakfast	Lunch	Dinner
Sunday	<u>Pancakes</u> Served with a choice of fruit topping.	<u>Sandwiches</u> Filling of choice such as ham or cheese.	<u>Roast</u> Roasted sweet potato, vegetables and a side of meat/protein.

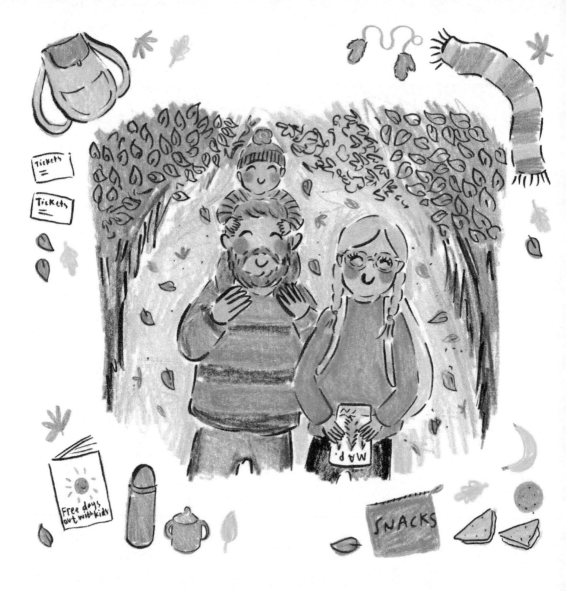

24. eXcursions

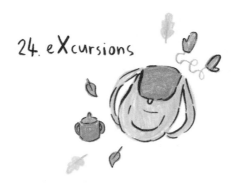

Okay, I was always going to struggle with a relevant word that actually starts with the letter 'x' but this is a good topic worth covering so stick with me. This chapter is about all things day trips and how to be as prepared as you possibly can. What to pack, where to go, and in general how to survive! When you've got a baby the times of being spontaneous and just turning up to places have gone, but that doesn't mean you can't get out and about and have fun. It just means being organised and one step ahead wherever possible.

Here is a useful checklist:

Tick	Item(s)
❏	Always find out how long it'll take to get there, including accounting for traffic.
❏	Check if booking in advance is an option, as sometimes this can save a long queue on arrival.
❏	Have spare change for the car park.
❏	An essential first aid kit can never be a bad thing to have with you- think plasters and medicine sachets.
❏	Take a packed lunch (for the adults too) so you don't have to rely on finding somewhere suitable, and include snacks (tired and hungry grown ups are no fun either!)
❏	Pack nappies, wipes, spare baby grows, bibs, a no-spill sippy cup, muslins, and outfit changes for your little one (taking an additional layer in case the weather changes).
❏	Take a couple of toys/books for distraction, including something helpful for teething times.
❏	Have the pram rain cover to hand for all seasons, and sun cream for the summer.
❏	Take the pram, even if you're planning to use a carrier since the pram might come in handy for a nap.
❏	If you've made it through chapter 16 you might want to consider a travel potty too!

eXcursions

That's a lot of things to consider for a simple day out, but it'll become second nature soon enough. If that list hasn't scared you off, then here are some considerations when deciding where to go:

The zoo is a family excursion that usually springs to mind, and whilst it is lovely to learn about animals by meeting them face to face, have you considered a farm or animal sanctuary instead? Zoo's can be quite unnatural and restrictive places for animals taken away from their natural habitats for the purpose of money making. Whereas animal sanctuaries provide more of a peaceful, natural environment and are often run as charities. Which, let's face it, is not just good for the animals but it also offers your little one a greater understanding when it comes to caring for our four legged friends.

Local parks or hiking trails as well as trips to the seaside are some more great ways of teaching the next generation about the great outdoors, and for an indoors option consider a trip to a museum for a potentially low-no cost entry.

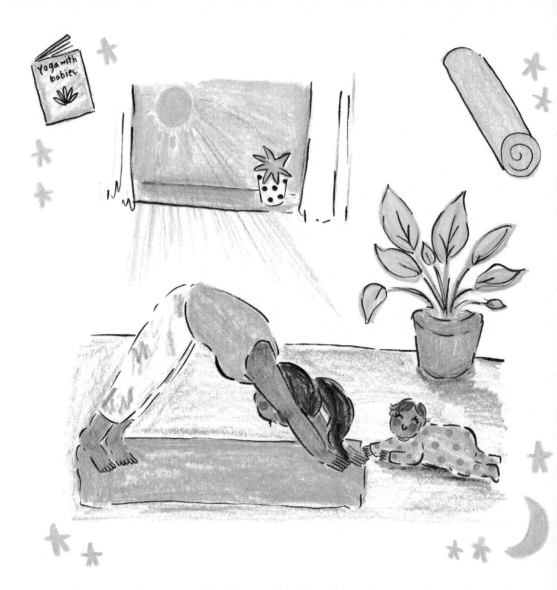

25. Yoga

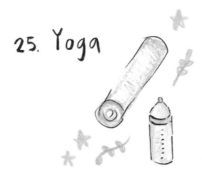

If you read the 'About Me' section at the start of this book, you'll know that I am into yoga. I have practised for years and also completed a 3 year teaching qualification with the British Wheel of Yoga. So of course the 'Y' chapter in this book was always going to be about yoga! In particular, this chapter covers a few considerations to make if you are interested in practising yoga after giving birth, whilst also offering some information on baby yoga. I hope some of it is helpful, but as with all chapters in this book if this one isn't your thing, skip to the next!

The most important message to convey here is to take time to pause after giving birth. Not only should the first month be a time for you to recuperate and adjust, your body really needs time to physically recover. I won't go into the details too much because it would create another book, but essentially your pelvic floor will have either been stretched a lot, cut, torn apart, or it could be completely intact but you'll have undergone major abdominal surgery, or have diastasis recti (separated abdominal muscles). Either way, you don't have the same body you had before or during pregnancy so it's especially important to listen to this new body and tune into its needs. As well as taking its toll physically, having a baby is a hugely emotional time. Give yourself permission to acknowledge that this is normal, you've gained intense responsibility during a time when there are hormones flowing through your body and which will continue to do so for several more months if you are breastfeeding.

Based on this, the advice from doctors and also midwives is to wait 6-8 weeks before practising yoga at all. If you had an epidural this may stay in your system for a lot longer so do be mindful of this, and there will also be high levels of the relaxin hormone in your body which increases flexibility to a point of risking injury when practising yoga. So adapt your practice with care and caution, and let your teacher know you have had a baby so they can offer suitable modifications for you. Personally, it took me 9 months to get back into a yoga studio. Of course I could have gone earlier but I was exhausted from sleep deprivation, I had anxiety about leaving Sienna, and then when I was able to leave her I was quite restricted in terms of childcare options. This is where mum and baby yoga can be great.

Taking your baby with you to yoga won't offer you the same level of relaxation at the end of the class as if you went alone, so we can't really compare the two as a like for like. However, I do recommend looking for local mum and baby yoga classes. As with all baby groups you have the bonus of meeting other mums and babies whilst giving your little one a boost of confidence when it comes to their social skills, but what's really great about baby yoga is that there are heaps of health benefits for your baby. These include relieving colic and wind, stimulating brain development, and boosting their immune system as well as the emotional benefits associated with the bonding element of practising yoga with you.

If you are still keen to practice yoga yourself but can't get to a class then maybe home practice is for you. Providing you have been medically cleared to do so, here are some postures I'd recommend to ease you back into a regular practice. Sometimes it can be a little overwhelming when thinking of allocating the time and energy for a whole 20-30 minutes of practice when your resources are already so depleted, so how about 1 posture a week to begin with, or just 5 minutes whenever you can:

Asana (Posture)	Instructions/Information	Benefits
Balasana (child's pose)	Aim to settle into this one for 5 minutes, 10 if you can. Ease into it from all fours sending your hips back to your heels. Your knees can be together, or about mat-width apart- but the idea is to arrive at a place of comfort so if it feels right then forget trying to replicate how it's meant to 'look'. Arms alongside your body (or out in front for an extended child's pose). When you're there, breathe. Take full breaths expanding throughout your whole body, front and back. Enjoy a rare moment's peace and allow your mind to float off into the mat (or pillow) with your head.	This pose helps to release your neck and upper back, while loosening stiff hips and offering a gentle stretch to your lower back and glutes. But most importantly, it's a stress reliever!

Asana (Posture)	Instructions/Information	Benefits
Gomukhasana (cow face pose)- arms only	From a seated position, you essentially want to hold your hands together behind your back but with one elbow pointing up and one pointing down. If your hands don't meet you can use a strap or more realistically, a muslin or tea towel which will probably be more available to you and will work just fine for you to hold onto behind your back. Keep your head and neck neutral (I find I have to almost tuck my chin in to avoid it naturally rising up). Hold the position for five deep breaths, release, and repeat to the other side.	This one is really useful for those neck and shoulder aches after sitting a little hunched to feed your baby (applies to both breastfeeding and bottle-feeding).

Asana (Posture)	Instructions/Information	Benefits
Viparita Karani (legs up the wall)	Find some space next to a wall, where you'll feel safe to lie. Consider using a folded blanket or a pillow which would align with where your lower back ends up on the mat when your bum is next to the wall. Take your legs up the wall either straight or bent- however it feels comfortable for you. Take breaks and if it feels too much to have the legs extended you can lower them by bringing your feet together and taking the knees out wide but closer to your body. Settle into this one for around 5 minutes or as long as feels comfortable, and allow each breath to take you deeper into a place of rest.	By elevating your legs this pose helps to relieve swelling around the ankles and feet which can be fairly common after having a baby. Even if you don't have this issue, the pose promotes recirculation in general, and relieves tension in the legs and feet, whilst balancing the nervous system. Name a new mum who doesn't need to feel more balanced?!

Asana (Posture)	Instructions/Information	Benefits
Adho mukha svanasana (downward dog)	Starting on all fours, tuck your toes under before sending the hips back towards your heels and lifting your knees off the mat gradually. Lift your hips, lower your gaze and relax your head, neck and shoulders. Be kind to yourself in the knowledge that your glutes and hamstrings will be tight as a result of balancing your growing baby bump during pregnancy. When in position, you might find it nice to cycle out the legs to help add warmth into the hamstrings and add a little extra stretch for your calf muscles. Hold this pose for 15-30 seconds, breathing steadily before lowering back onto your knees on all fours. From here, why not treat yourself to a bonus child's pose for an element of relaxation.	Downward dog helps to strengthen your arms and shoulders, which are important areas to keep strong for feeding your baby. The pose also increases blood flow to your brain which has added benefits of boosting mood, great for those down days.

Asana (Posture)	Instructions/Information	Benefits
Virabhadrasana I (Warrior 1)	All parents are warriors, and this pose will have you feeling like it. From standing, step back with one foot and turn that foot out at around a 45 degree angle. Bend your front knee (keeping the knee in line with your ankle so you don't overshoot it), and keep your hips facing forwards. Take your arms up and overhead (palms of the hands facing each other), rounding the shoulders back and down to release the usual tension points. Breathe through this Warrior 1 pose for 5 slow breaths, or however many you feel able to before switching sides and repeating it equally.	Warriors are all about strength and so it's no surprise that this pose helps to build strength as well as stability, and endurance. Standing tall in Warrior 1 increases your circulation, helping to create that all important energy we often feel lacking as a new parent.

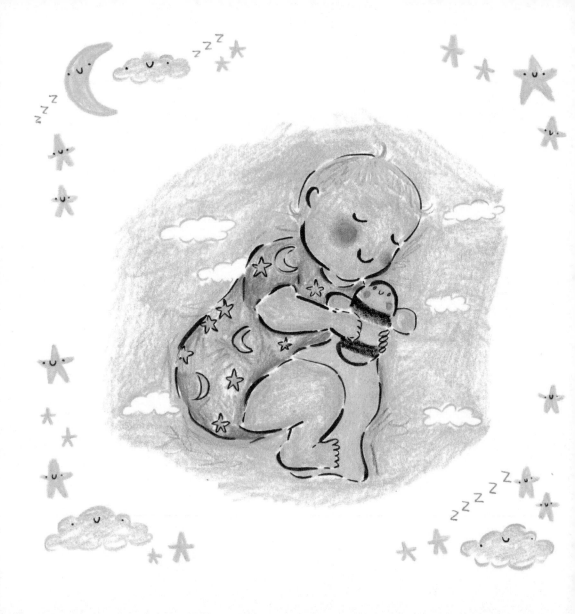

26. Zzz

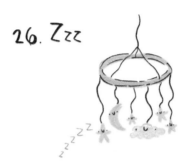

We covered sleep to a certain extent in the first chapter but with this being the number one topic discussed by all parents, it's only right that we come full circle. In chapter 1, we covered wake windows and how following these timeframes of recommended awake hours can help to guide your baby into a good rhythm. Now we learn more about sleep science, because sometimes there is a lot more to it than we might realise. I'm not one for sleep training in the sense of the cry it out or extinction method, and I'm not a particularly huge fan of the word 'training' since I believe there is an element of developmental readiness when it comes to sleep that absolutely differs amongst all babies. However, what I have come to realise is that we help our babies to do and learn so many things, so it makes sense that we can help with sleep. We can show them how to bang two shapes together and teach them the words 'bang bang' which they soon start to associate with the action for example. Sleep is slightly different, since we can't directly teach them by demonstration but bear with me because I am going somewhere with this point! Quite often it can seem as if we have followed the same routine day in and day out, the same awake windows have been followed, yet some nights offer more sleep than others. This is where sleep science can help, with our sanity if nothing else, because we start to learn how, why and when babies sleep. We also learn that sometimes the broken sleep is normal for the stage they are going through, and sometimes we can't do anything different to change it. Doing something different can actually make the association with sleep change, which in turn could have a negative impact. So there are times when you just have to ride it out with reassurance in knowing that it's probably just a phase.

What we do know, is that when your baby is around 9-10 months old they start to recognise sequences of events. This means they begin to associate actions with each other. For instance, they may start to grab the spoon for themselves during meal times and try to put it in their mouth, or they might start pointing at things to indicate what they want and then start moving in that direction to build the sequence between where they are and where they want to be. Useful to know, but what does this have to do with sleep? I've rambled a little here but with good intention. What I'm getting at, is that at this age we can help our babies to sleep in a similar way, by building a sequence of events that will lead up to their bedtime. From the age of about 4 months I'd read a book with Sienna in her nursery, give her a bath, and then give her a little massage before bed. Not being one for good sleep at night, when she started sleeping a little better (at times) from 10 months, it made perfect sense to me that she now understood the sequence. I'd changed nothing about our routine, so it was just that she could now associate this chain of events with bedtime. She was developmentally ready to sleep, and I was able to help her to learn that this time was approaching each day by following a simple routine. By the time she was 12 months she really understood words, I was also able to say things like 'sleep' which would follow with her putting her head down on the mattress, floor, sofa or wherever we were. I was then able to move away from feeding to sleep and implement a very gradual retreat from her nursery.

Sometimes sleep can be something we stress about with a baby, understandably so since being deprived of sleep is so hard. I hope that this chapter offers some reassurance in knowing that it is ok to ride this phase out without implementing drastic measures. As I have said time and time again within this book, every baby is different. So whilst the perspective I am writing with comes from my experiences through Sienna, I have supplemented this with extensive research and many conversations with other mums and subject matter experts. Of course if you are concerned about your little ones sleep from a health and wellbeing perspective, always seek advice from a health professional. Otherwise just prepare yourself for sleep to settle out when your baby is developmentally ready, through following awake windows (chapter 1) and implementing a strong routine. I hope that knowing there is light at the end of the tunnel will put your mind at ease.

Conclusion

I told you there was a lot of stuff! Whether you've been reading this on the go, picking chapters as and when you needed to know, or if you've just learnt the whole alphabet in preparation of your little one's arrival, well done for making it to the end! I say end, let's be honest- this is where it really begins!

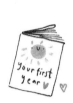

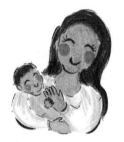

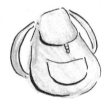

The A-Z of Parenting: Babies

Printed in Great Britain
by Amazon

15424782R00095